In the game of life,

who loves the most—wins!

Love, Wisdom & Healing

Todd Puntolillo

Dream Maker Productions
Margate, Florida

ISBN: 978-0-7596-7899-6 (sc)
ISBN: 978-0-7596-7898-9 (e)

Print information available on the last page.

www.wisdomandhealing.com

1stBooks - rev. 11/10/2021

Contents

Part 3. Delving

Part 4. The Tools

Dedication

I dedicate this book to truth-seekers everywhere. Letting go of the past, we advance into the higher realm of possibilities...

The Kingdom Within.

My special gratitude to numerous individuals and groups who offered the spiritual encouragement I required to stay on my path: the late Grace V. Dickinson, C.S.B., a teacher who taught Truth by living and demonstrating it; Rev. Barbara Lunde of the Science of Mind Center of Boca Raton, Florida, who taught me how to think rather than just what to think; and Valerie Quinlan, who coached me to find the beauty of the unseen world of energy and to be more than I knew I could be.

I also wish to acknowledge many speakers, writers, and teachers, past and present, who have inspired me and pointed the way. Their teachings have brought me to a place where I have learned to see through new eyes and to live and write from my heart.

Thanks to these people, my family, and friends for helping to write the story of my life.

Foreword

The poem that follows tells where I stood in 1975, a conscientious but still naive young man watching his world crumble around him. It is often sad and painful to see what we must put ourselves through before we can finally become teachable. The most important lesson I had to learn was to stop looking outside of myself for Truth. It was time to stop labeling people and experiences and putting them into tidy boxes on well-organized shelves. Life was to be lived with open eyes and a willing heart. That low point, when I wrote "Freedom's Way," was the beginning of my new life. I now smile when looking back at it.

No book can give you all the answers, but somewhere in the symbolism that follows, if you really want it, are many of the keys to a joyous and fulfilling life. On every page you will find ideas, many of which you may never have heard presented in just this way. As you read, and possibly reread, *The Dream Maker*, you can find more than one hundred concepts that I used to construct Part 1 of this book.

The "Dream Maker" is a name I use to describe spiritual consciousness. The character represents the wisdom within us, our Higher Self. Our inner wisdom will lead us only as far as the chains we have chosen will allow. When we gain enough courage to remove them, there will be no limit to our joy and possibilities!

This book is presented in four parts. Part 1, "The Dream Maker," is allegorical. It presents its information in a way that will make you pause and ask yourself poignant questions.

Part 2, "Short Stories," are a sampling of four years of writing for *The Happy Times Monthly*, an all-good-news newspaper based in Boca Raton, Florida. These are quick, easy-to-read commentaries on everyday life and expand the information from Part 1.

Part 3, "Delving," is a different kind of writing, somewhat lyrical and full of fancy. Included are some biographical sketches. It offers a deeply spiritual approach, whereas Parts 1 and 2 are a little more pragmatic.

Part 4, "The Tools," is a guide to building the kind of consciousness that will empower you. It contains the basic mind tools for designing a life. It explains in greater detail what energy and consciousness are and how to use them.

All in all, this should be a fun-filled, easy-to-read book that will enable you to find the peace, joy, and power that have always existed within you. Happy reading!

Todd Puntolillo

Freedom's Way

The darkness closed in on me;
the prison doors clanged tight.
My eyes with tears were brimming.
Life seemed a losing fight.
When I was just an infant the tragedy began.
My elders demanded things just right,
to be a proper man.
The shackles they put on me
are those that they still wear.
It's how the world manipulates
and acts as if it cares.

In school I learned to read and write
and never to do wrong;
Salute the flag, and pray to God,
and sing a marching song.
I tried to give my love to all
and stand up brave and bold,
But "That's not how it's done,"
is what I, then, was told.
"You must not touch, nor speak, nor show,
your feelings you must hide.
Once they're let out you'll be put down,
so lock them deep inside."

I followed life's strange standards
and therefore never found...
what really makes a happy man

or makes the saddest sound.
I yearned to meet true people
and touch their very soul,
But for convention's sake I wed
and lived a normal role.
And then I worked to pay the bills
and paid the bills to live.
I gave my all, with thanks from none,
so I really didn't give.

I'd been locked in so very long;
all outlets had been plugged.
The whole routine and dreary scene
had really got me drugged.

I now stand at the crisis point,
the decision I shall make,
will set me free to live and give,
I know it's no mistake.
I've lived and loved to no avail,
but while my heart still beats,
I'll choose my life and freedom,
my wins and my defeats.

The doors will now swing open,
I'll give my every all
to see and hear, to touch and feel
and follow freedom's call.
For I love God's creation, in love I will invest,
'Cause life is all that I can have ...
...and Freedom's Way is best!

Todd Puntolillo 1975

Part 1

The Dream Maker

*An allegorical tale, dedicated to enhanced
values and the manifestation
of a greater peace,
love and happiness.*

The Little Man

I settled into my aisle seat, fastened my seat belt, and brought my seat back into its full upright position. It is my custom, when flying, to select an aisle seat as far forward as possible, so that I might be one of the first passengers off the plane and down to the rental car counter. I learned a lot about how to get the most out of my business hours. Uncharacteristically, today my mind was not on the business at hand. I had experienced several setbacks and, with introspection and retrospection, was wondering if I was running my life, or if my life was running me. As I sat there pondering my worries, disappointments, and prospects, I suddenly became aware of the person in the seat next to me. I didn't see or hear him— I just felt his presence. I looked to my right and there sat an elderly man. He didn't look like much. His clothing was loose-fitting and ordinary. He wore no jewelry, not even a watch. He obviously wasn't a businessman. His face had such a radiant glow that, as he smiled at me, I just couldn't help reaching out to shake his hand and introduce myself. His eyes sparkled, exuding a youthful impishness. I was certain that this man didn't have deadlines, cares, pressures, and worries like me.

He spoke, "You have many concerns, my son, but I'll let you in on a little-known statistic. Ninety percent of all those problems you are letting eat at you will never occur. I offer this: You can't be grateful and unhappy at the same time."

"You can tell I'm worried?" I asked, taken completely off guard. "What about the other ten percent?"

He continued, "You can handle the other ten percent. Life would be meaningless without some obstacles. Your brain is a computer. You input data and it sorts, files, and retrieves until you find a suitable answer. If logic isn't enough, you can call on your subconscious and tap into your intuition. The *thinker*, the real you, that operates your brain and body can supply your every need, even if your answer has to come from the ends of the earth.

"Problems aren't all tragedies; *they are merely unresolved questions!* Consider this: If you don't feed your subconscious with high expectations, purpose, and wholesome concepts, it will immediately dig up an old problem you have left unresolved and enroll you, through your feelings, to deal with it—whether you want to or not. You need challenges to grow and you need to *give*, *receive*, *share*, and *grow* to be happy and fulfilled."

"Receiving? Isn't that selfish?" I queried.

"Receiving can be joyful, but some folks try to receive only and not to give. Others are givers and feel too embarrassed or unworthy to receive. It is necessary to do both—you can't only inhale or only exhale. The beautiful cyclical nature of life is give and take, ebb and flow."

"You seem to know all about happiness," I suggested. "You know what I wish ...?"

Before I could finish, he looked at me quite startled and exclaimed, "Then you know! I can't figure out how you recognized me, but I guess it's time to pay up."

"Pay up?" I asked.

"When you recognize the *Dream Maker*, you get three wishes. *I must warn you, however, I don't have to grant them.*"

"Oh no!" I said without thinking. "I didn't recognize you. ... I was just, well, sort of..."

"Well," he chuckled, "maybe I jumped the gun, but now that I've agreed to give you three wishes, and you were half-started making a wish when I interrupted, go ahead and wish away!"

The Wishes

I was flabbergasted! Who was this guy? I had never heard of the *Dream Maker*. "Am I going to pour out my heart to some character from a Loony-Tunes production," I wondered, "or is he a sage, a wise man, or a prophet? Perhaps he's a genie, or a master trained in Tibet, or a guru ..." Well, whatever was happening, I couldn't chance letting this opportunity slip through my fingers. Unable to help myself, I blurted, "You can grant three wishes? You're kidding! You're not kidding?"

He waited patiently for me to stop rambling; then with knowing eyes, he spoke. "I don't really grant wishes. Wishes are weak, whining expressions of doubt uttered by a person who isn't willing to work for what he believes and wants. Give me instead your three requests. Ask."

There was a long silence as I sorted through the events of the past few moments. I don't know how long this took, but as I glanced around, I noticed that we were above the clouds and I hadn't even been aware of taking off. I can't remember ever being so preoccupied.

I dreamed of riches, a fine home, and a yacht. I had seen many things in life to be coveted, but to this time, I never saw any *thing* that couldn't be taken away or lost. As a matter of fact, most things that I had received, without proper preparation or without earning them, disappeared as quickly as they had appeared. The truth is— everything I own draws energy from me in the form of work, worry, or expense. I had to think clearly. I didn't want to waste a *request*.

The First Request

It was time for the "what-if " syndrome. What if he's a phoney? What if I make a mistake? What if I am making a fool of myself? I thought about the ninety percent of my worries that will never occur and slowly began to evolve new "what ifs," such as: What if there are possibilities that I have never considered? What if I can make choices that will redirect my life? What if this was *that momentous occasion I've been waiting for all my life*—that big moment when I shed my cocoon and spread my wings?

I took a deep breath. "**Wisdom**," I said. "If I could only understand life, my place in it, and the laws that govern the universe, I could stop swimming against the current. I could flow with the energy of Life—I would be happy, prosperous, and peaceful."

The little man closed his eyes, then nodded. He fixed his gaze on my eyes and never uttered a word. I took the cue and proceeded to consider my second request.

The Second Request

I was hoping that my first request had already been granted. If it had, and if he could, I wouldn't be so likely to make a mistake with my next two. I felt myself tightening up. I was becoming anxious, doubtful, and worried about the outcome. How often I had worried my way through events I had deemed important. It seemed to me that my main source of torture in life was *worry*. What request could I make that would end this self-inflicted misery?

All of a sudden it dawned on me. I was clear. "**Faith**," I told him. "If I can know and believe that Life is *for* me, that I have a right to be creative and happy, there would be nothing to worry about. The outcome would be a blessing for all concerned."

In the past I had worried, so of course now I worried. In the past I mistrusted, so now I was mistrusting. I could think of story after story from my past—always in my past, that seemed to disable me. I must now throw caution to the wind and start thinking into the future. I could no longer let old stories determine what my future held for me. I felt an upsurge from within. Ideas and ideals were welling up inside of me.

Famed author and endocrinologist, Deepak Chopra, said that we think sixty thousand thoughts each day and about ninety-five percent of them are the same thoughts we thought about yesterday. It seemed to me that thinking from the past had closed off my possibilities for a future, and now the time had come for me to make the decisions that would change my life forever.

I told him of my insight. He smiled and replied, "There is no power nor possibility in the past. We are not our stories. We just use these stories so that we can be victims. As victims we don't need to take responsibility for our lives. We can make excuses instead. To take responsibility for one's life is to accept the fact that we are where we are because of what we believed in the past. Most importantly, we can be what we would be by creating new possibilities, making new choices, and changing our focus from blame and criticism to acceptance of that which is and expectancy of what can be.

"Every thought and action has a consequence. The consequence is not optional. You wrote the story of your past. You are now writing your future. There is only one common denominator in every situation you have ever encountered. It is that you were there. The power of your word to create is absolute! If your word goes out into the Universe and attracts what you are believing, as many have come to learn, you must make sure that your word blesses all, because therein lies its power."

"Tell me, Mr. Dream Maker," I asked, "how does one *put forth his word?*"

"Some people pray," he responded, "but when prayer has been unfruitful, it is because people focus on the problem and beg what they believe to be an absentee deity whom they don't trust. This, my friend, affords little hope.

"Powerful prayer, including affirmations and visualization, is centering oneself in silence, focusing on your oneness with the all-inclusive, creative Mind, trusting the power of your word, and declaring your vision of health, prosperity, and wholesome relationships into the Universe—within. Then, silently listening. Finally, releasing one's word peacefully, expecting good. Sometimes patience is needed; other times, results are immediate. Always the word, backed with conviction, desire, and integrity, attracts to you all the good you can envision. It is a conversation with the Creator where you speak or write your word, then meditate (listen), and, finally, let it go and trust. Eventually, this process becomes automatic and abbreviates itself to envisioning and trusting. The ultimate communication is silent oneness."

I was so pleased with myself. I had reached deeply within and two answers had come to me about which I felt very good. I looked at my new friend. Again he silently nodded, then refocused his gaze into my eyes.

By this time I didn't feel like some kid wishing. Instead, I felt confident. I was certain that I was going to get what I requested.

"Now," I pondered, "that was the easy part." The first two requests took much less courage than the third and last. This was the time to decide whether I should ask for something more selfish—something just for me. It would be only one of three. Maybe a pot of gold, or a Rolls Royce, a mansion, or the chance to play shortstop for the Mets...

The Third Request

There came a cold feeling over me. I imagined myself first in a forty-room mansion, then driving back and forth in my Rolls Royce, then sitting at a table counting and recounting my pieces of gold. I saw myself as a hermit, then as a multimillionaire with an entourage of servants, PR men, bodyguards, and financial managers jealously running my affairs. I experienced, in my mind, people coming around in hopes of getting my money.

I was stopped—frozen between fear and lack of commitment. *"I don't know what I want! I have no real purpose in life. I flit like a butterfly from flower to flower, dodging sprinklers and flying into walls. I don't have meaning, just action. I'm a dust chaser, a paper shuffler, and a grass cutter trying to maintain, and frankly, the older I get, the more ground I lose."*

"To whom or what do you attribute this?" he asked.

"My parents' programming, my bosses' demands, my wife's agenda, my children's needs..." I paused.

"Victim?" He chuckled. "You have turned your life and theirs over to whim and fancy. You have disempowered them with blame. The only consequence of disempowering others is to disempower yourself. You don't really make your-self right by making them wrong. You just take away the possibility of creating a better future when you make these stories the reality of your life while you remain chained to your victim (no possibility) consciousness.

"You believe you've sinned or that some-one has sinned against you. Originally, the word sin was an archer's term meaning 'to miss the mark.' Repent has as its root, *penser*, to think. So repent means rethink. Here's the new version of sin and repentance: If you sin (miss the mark), try repentance (rethinking). Chances are, miss-ing the mark in the first place was a failure to think. Doesn't this lighten up the sin, guilt, and repentance story a bit? *If you want to be enlight-ened—lighten up!*"

"I think I've got it!" I exclaimed. "I want to give and receive **unconditional love**. Unquali-fied love is the nature of the Creator of all life, and all subsequent creation. My happiest moments are spent sharing love. My third request is to be loving and loved."

The Question

"Noble requests," the Dream Maker remarked. "Noble and powerful. *But one thing is still lacking.*"

"Lacking?" I repeated. I was stumped. I stared back at him with a helpless, blank expression. "If I had asked for *things*, I would have made myself vulnerable to weakness of character. Necessity creates, ease vegetates," I mumbled as if it were a maxim. "If I had wisdom, faith, and love, I could be happy, harmless, and useful. What could possibly be lacking?"

He spoke calmly and softly, "In a moment. First, understand that happiness, as an effect, is dependent upon external events. Take away the required conditions and happiness disappears. *Serenity*, on the other hand, is the state of being peaceful and content *regardless* of outward conditions. It is an inner knowing of one's completeness and intrinsic perfection. Serenity comes when you stop fearfully *reacting* to each story that comes your way and begin to *respond*, with trust, to the Power of the Universe that lives within you. When committed to your life's purpose, walls come down and peace ensues. Like the tiny acorn containing everything it needs to become a huge oak tree, you arrived here with a purpose. Knowing you were born with the blueprint to achieve your purpose opens the door to the peace and serenity that has always resided within you. Look no further, your bliss comes from a loving, trusting heart."

"Your First Choice...

Wisdom. A well-thought-out request. Most of life's problems are the direct result of making wrong decisions. Everyone is one hundred percent responsible for choosing his own thoughts. Our thinking determines our experience. *This is the Law, and here is the formula*: The Great Origin and Cause 'thinks' (expresses). These thoughts/expressions are pure energy. This energy transforms into color, form, and substance by means of variation in electrical frequency or, more concisely, vibration. We call substance matter. Matter, by human definition, is limited to dimensions, weight, and density. *The substance of creation, however, is limitless energy*.

"**Here is how we make this Law work in our lives:** *We choose beliefs, whether positive or negative, which eventually are expressed as outward manifestations. Every choice we make manifests. The substance of these manifestations is thought-energy. The source of our every need is the unlimited Intelligence of the Universe. Every experience in life is a transaction of Mind, and every thought moves energy*.

"By virtue of your divine nature as the expression of spiritually creative thought-energy, you include wisdom (collective intelligence) as

17

a component of your being. To be wise, simply access the infinite field of intelligence through *wise intention and meditative contemplation.*

"The Universe, Cosmic Power, or however we choose to identify the Creator of all intelligence, life, law, and truth, created everything out of nothing—except itself. Whatever *stuff* it is that the Creator is, composes us.

"Everything that exists, from the mathematics of infinity and eternality, is One. We may be distinct from one another but never separate. To put someone else down is to shoot one's own foot. We can't hide our untruths. We can't avoid life. We're just hanging out there for all the world to see, and every thought and action creates consequences.

"When we help another we bless ourselves. To give makes us richer. To enliven another gives us life. It is Law, it is unavoidable, and it now exists within your consciousness; therefore, it is undeniably yours. By creating wisdom as a purpose in life, you have opened yourself to its flow. Your first request is granted. Having sought wisdom externally, you have found it within."

"Your Second Choice...

Faith. The book of Hebrews reads, 'Now faith is the substance of things hoped for, the evidence of things not seen.' How difficult it is for us to have faith without understanding. If you thought that a man at your door late at night was carrying a gun, you would be terrified. If, however, he showed you that it was a cellular telephone, you would stop being afraid. When you *understand* the truth, it is much easier to have faith.*

"Right now you can know that you are protected, and will prosper, by spiritual and natural laws. Your Creator, although not human, is your Father and

---

*Important note: The statement about mistaking a cellular phone for a gun is not nearly as farfetched as it might sound. A number of years ago I arrived early in the morning at a diner where I was to meet my associate, Ted. I was dressed in a dark pin-striped suit and driving a black Ford. I noticed a strange young man wearing a karate outfit watching me, but had no idea why. Ted was late, so I decided to check with my answering machine to see if he left me a message. I went to the pay phone, dialed, and pulled out my little black remote device to access my messages. The karate guy watched and looked extremely alarmed.

Unable to reach Ted, I went and sat in my Crown Vic and waited. A few minutes later there was a tap on my window. Two policemen stood there *with guns drawn*. I opened the window and they asked me if I was armed. I told them that I wasn't. They asked why I was there. I told them. They explained about a call they had received identifying me as an assassin with a detonator. I laughed and showed them my remote. I then mentioned the strange guy in the karate ghi. A knowing look came over their faces and, without even asking me for identification or any search, they turned their backs to me and went inside the diner.

Mother. Your inheritance of the masculine (outreaching, protective, principled) and feminine (attracting, intuitive, loving) qualities of your Source makes you a complete being, including unlimited possibilities and actualities. Your need to express your masculinity and femininity, regardless of your gender, is normal. Strength and love are not roles, but rather the combined nature of all beings. Affirmation of truth focuses the Law and produces the desired result. Faith avails much. Simple trust in the Power within you is omnipotent. Remember, *'Doubt never produced a useful result.'*

"I see by the look on your face that you have glimpsed possibilities. Those thoughts, over which you were agonizing when we met, have been dissipated. You have an understanding, the basis for faith. Build on this foundation."

They returned in a few minutes with the strange guy in handcuffs! He was on the run and self-convicted by his paranoia.

This is an example of how we create our own truth and live under our own illusions, often suffering the results of an event that never occurred. The facts, circumstances, or seeming conditions are not always truth. This is how Truth can triumph over apparent "reality" and therefore make conditions or circumstances change. By Truth's mere realization, illusion dissipates. We call the process "healing" or "miraculous." It is not as much a miracle as a Divine Law being unveiled. When a light suddenly shines in the darkness, the darkness disappears and all that exists is the light. Nothing actually changes in this process. It is more like an awakening. That, by the way, is the purpose of this book: to create an awakening of the Truth within that has always existed...in spite of the illusions that encompass us all.

Money

I was speechless. This person, this enlightened being, was beaming like a man with purpose. He spoke enthusiastically, "I know you considered wealth. Why did you not ask for money?"

I told him, "I almost asked for money. I have spent my whole life chasing the 'Dollar Bill.' To have money would give me time to pursue something nobler. However, it is not more time that I need; it is a higher quality of life. To have the virtues I requested would make me happy, and if happiness is not what I am really seeking, what is? I decided that money was temporal and therefore inferior."

"Happiness," he said, "is not about getting, it is about being. Don't seek happiness—*be happy*. If you wait for events to occur in order to be happy, your life will be confusing and disappointing. Money may not be your first priority," he added, "but it is not evil. It is, in fact, neutral—meaningless. There is nothing wrong with money. It is to the businessman what crops are to the farmer and fish to the fisherman. Money is a means of exchange. Your supply of money is limited only by the amount of useful ideas you implement and services you render or cause to be rendered. The desire to acquire money is not evil. *An all-consuming lust for money is a horrible waste of your life.* Falsely empowering money as the Universal cure-all is laughable. But *the biggest error is to live one's life in fear of being without money.* Stinginess and the fear of poverty are tragedies that throw one's thinking out of balance with the Universal Law, which declares to all, 'Give richly and you will receive richly.'"

He continued, "My son, you are never separated from your real Source. Enjoy money, respect it, use it, share it, give it, circulate it, bless and support it in your thoughts. Earn it ethically. It symbolizes growth, activity, the power to build, abundance, and a host of virtuous ideals. No one can deplete the Infinite. Never fear that there isn't enough for everybody.

"Mind always creates out of infinity. We cannot put a limit on the creative action of Mind. If we use our ability to create, by using the same process we spoke of before—thought converting energy to form—the Law will bring abundance of good, including money, into our lives. Wealth is the by-product of self-worth and expectancy. If we believe ourselves worthy, remove the barriers of hatred and resentment, love what money truly represents, and maintain our faith in Universal Abundance, we can always expect our every need to be met without a struggle. You can see, a struggle represents a refusal to trust the Power within.

"We don't resent electricity just because someone used it destructively. Electricity has advanced mankind and brought conveniences to our lives. The misdirection of its power doesn't make electricity or money evil. Recognize money for the good it symbolizes and the wonderful convenience of exchange for which it was intended."

"Your Third Choice..."

He was interrupted by the pilot over the intercom. We were beginning our descent and would be landing soon.

"**Love** is the core of all creation. If only one word could describe the Parent of a universe and its laws, the word could only be Love. To believe that the world, as we know it, evolved accidentally, by means of some microscopic organisms, is like believing that a skyscraper accidentally evolved from a rock pile. No coincidence can explain creation. *Nothing happens without Intelligence.* Mind is the source of all creation and the nature of the Creative Mind is Love."

"What about atheists?" I interjected. This was something I couldn't fathom and it had plagued me from youth. How can there be a creation without a creator?

"Atheists are people who don't believe in *their own concept of God.* They believe in Nature, Truth, Love, or Law. What they don't believe in is a mystical being making life and death decisions over a world full of helpless victims. *I don't believe in that kind of God*, but that doesn't make me an atheist."

He returned to his subject, "Your desire to love unconditionally will be rewarded. Keep this goal always before you and realize the importance of loving yourself, because you cannot love anyone else truly unless you restore your own self-worth. To progress, guilt and self-hatred must be released. Behold the nature of love, for it is the real you. The Universal Creator, out of which everything was formed, is within everyone and everything you see."

I really had to think about that.

"Your next step is to release and forgive people who have, in your opinion, wronged or threatened you. Recognize that these people are acting out their lives as victims of teachings of other victims. They are your teachers. Learn from them, but don't imitate them. Be authentic! Loving is letting go and trusting. Let go, my friend, and be Love expressed. You can readily see that Love isn't something I can give you. The more I try to give it away, the more I have. Love is an unlimited resource. If unconditional love is your goal, I suggest you start by giving it away.

"Be clear, do not accept abuse from others, nor condone evil or cruel acts. Although you must love the spiritual core of everyone, it is not necessary for them to sit in your soup. Mentally, and if necessary physically, free yourself and release them into a loving Universe. You can rise no higher than that which you believe to be true about others. See perfection in others—not necessarily their actions, but, rather, their spiritual, intrinsic worth. In proportion to your ability to see the good in all creation, in that proportion will your consciousness be raised and your understanding of love be demonstrated."

About That One Thing Lacking...

"Love without **discipline** is like a beautiful automobile locked in a garage. It is great to have, but unless you get it started, you're going nowhere. Discipline is the element you must add to Wisdom, Faith, and Love to make them a day-to-day reality. You could not have asked me for it because it is certainly the part of the job that you must accomplish for yourself. It means patience and persistence. *To make your world, and everyone else's, a wonderful place to be, use the energy of desire, enthusiasm, determination, disciplined right thinking, trusting, affirming, refocusing, and envisioning as your daily practice.*"

Touchdown

I thanked him profusely for sharing his wisdom with me. I promised him I'd take time every morning to meditate and prepare myself to live fully the day at hand with gratitude. I vowed to read something inspirational before bed each night in order to feed my subconscious and let it digest its spiritual nourishment while I slept. This would be my discipline.

He persuaded me to practice wisdom, faith, and love in my daily encounters in order to sharpen my spiritual skills and bring healing to my world.

Then and there I committed myself to share my new information with whomever might want to hear it.

"You have absorbed a great deal in a short time," he noted. "I want to share a few thoughts with you before we part. *Make them yours*.

"No one owns an idea. Ideas enrich us. If I give you a dollar and you give me a dollar, that exchange leaves us with one dollar each. If I give you an idea and you give me an idea, we each walk away with two ideas. Be in the 'exchange business'—share ideas.

"*Remember …*
There is always an answer.
The answer is always good.

There is not only one right answer.
Rightly understood, there are infinite
  viewpoints.
You are unlimited in possibility.
Think in grand terms.
There is Unity in all Life.
Love conquers all!
Forgiveness and gratitude are the secrets
  of an unfettered soul, youthful resil-
  ience, and a rich life.
Your greater or lesser ability to demon-
  strate Divine Laws depends upon your
  willingness to exchange limited beliefs
  for unlimited Truth.
The Law of Attraction will bring every-
  thing you ever need to your doorstep.
Stand by your truth, expect good, and
  then stand by the door and open it to
the Universal Flow!
Expectancy of good is spiritual power.
Transcend your sense information. The
  five senses do not always report reality.
Develop a spiritual sense.
Meditate daily. Silently listen to the
  rhythm of life.
Visualize world peace, then be peaceful.
Action often precedes understanding;
  therefore, act as if you are spiritually
  whole—in this way you will make health
  and harmony your reality.
Your expression of good blesses Mankind.

Bestow peace and happiness on all whom
you mentally and physically embrace.
The most powerful healing formula is to
let go of your concerns and trust Life.
Praise God, praise yourself, praise others.
Avoid gossip and complaint; they are the
wrong use of your powerful word.
When you say 'I am' be sure to follow it
with something good. Your word attracts
exactly as you speak it. When you say
'I am' you are addressing the God-Self
within you.
Be grateful. Be happy. Love life. "

He smiled, turned, and walked away through the busy crowd. I watched as he disappeared from view.

As I walked through the airport, it was as though I were walking on clouds. I mused to myself, "I'll bet no matter what three requests I gave him, I would have left with the same message." The glow that he expressed was the Love he was being.

It is my hope that the next time you see that glow on someone's face, dear reader, it is when you look into your own mirror.

Part 2

Short Stories

Commentaries that will impact
the way you look
at life.

Subsequent Revelations

Back in 1988, while in a whimsical mood driving south to Miami, information started pouring into my mind. I had to pull over and write an outline because there was no way I could write anywhere near the speed that *The Dream Maker* flowed to me. The completion of the book was rapid, but subsequent revisions required study and contemplation.

The pages that follow have unfolded since the first publishing of *The Dream Maker*. It was a conscious choice on my part to write short, concise articles. Time seems to have accelerated. No one with whom I speak can understand how little free time seems available for the volumes of reading that most of us face daily.

Part 2 includes information to support the postulates of Part 1. I write the inspirational column for the *Happy Times Monthly*, an all-good-news newspaper, in Boca Raton, Florida. They answer such questions as: "Who am I?", "Why am I here?", and "What can I be doing while I'm here to be a part of the 'Grand Solution' currently in progress?" These were fun for me to write. I hope you enjoy them as much. Every page has a message. These messages are meant as tools to build a powerful healing philosophy.

Seeking the Cure

A child gleefully plays, screeching and laughing. A loud voice screams in retaliation, "Can't you be quiet and act your age?"

A housewife tells her husband, "I would like to open a flower shop. You know how good I am with gardening and plants." The husband replies, "You need money and business sense for that, and you don't have either."

Sometimes it comes across like this: "How many times do I have to show you the right way to do this?" The small print between the lines is louder than the words spoken. It says, "You are stupid." The further inference might be, "I'm intelligent and know the right way. You, however, don't have a clue. Without my directives, you are useless."

Most caring people would never call someone "useless" or "stupid," but many imply it without seeing the damage they are doing, usually to the ones they love the most. Without realizing that they are indirectly saying it, someone will imply "I am right. There is no room in my world for your opinions. For you to be right, I have to be wrong, and we know that can't happen!"

In order for many people to feel they are in control, they believe it is a requirement to lie to, manipulate, invalidate, and intimidate their *imagined* opponent. With this adversarial posture, is it any wonder that so many people have relationship problems ?

If I were given the power to cure just one ill that haunts mankind, I would pass up cancer, breeze by AIDS, and overlook heart disease *because curing the malady I have in mind might just cure most of the others as a side effect.*

The cure I would seek would be the cure for *criticism*. No disease shrivels up the souls of innocent children, destroys the family unit, ruins the business place, incapacitates government, nor produces stress like criticism. The terrible three (criticism, judgmentalism, and complaint) do more to dishearten the spirit and, in general, create misery, pain, and sorrow than anything else I have ever encountered. It is so commonplace that, in many cases, we don't even pause to take note when words of criticism are voiced. Sitcoms find their success in "put downs" while millions watch and laugh.

Criticism is so hideous that we even label criticism as "constructive" and "destructive" so we can invalidate someone and tell them that it is for their own good. Of course, there are times when we might share an opinion or offer a suggestion. This, however, can be done without "pointing the finger of guilt." I believe that criticism is always subjective and therefore the opinion of the criticizer, not absolute truth.

Do you ever feel like you work hard to make everyone around you happy and comfortable but receive no appreciation for your efforts? If you do, you are not alone. Millions go through life rarely being told how much their love and support mean to the ones their sacrifices benefit. The world is hungering for appreciation and praise. How seldom it is given. How precious it is! Tell those who support or serve you how much it means to you. It costs nothing and will pay big dividends—mutually. Recycle praise; it never gets old!

Although I don't have the cures, I do consider appreciation and praise to be antidotes. Here are some ingredients we can add to our formula: love, consideration, reason, communication, humbleness, awareness, gentleness, kindness, and patience. If people know that our feelings toward them are nurturing, they will help find common grounds to work things out. If we act like an adversary, we will be treated as one. As always, the choice is yours.

I decided to list the benefits of being critical, judgemental or just complaining so we all can take a deeper look at it. Please think deeply about "The Benefits of Criticism."

The Benefits of Criticism

- You get to watch people's face drop and spirit sink.
- You make it known that you are expressing a loveless soul.
- You get to teach children that they are inadequate or unlovable.
- You get to stunt the growth of a person who is struggling.
- You get to stop progress in the business enviroment.
- You get to undermine everyone around you.
- You get to create bad feelings wherever you go.
- You get to perpetuate racism and warlike thinking.
- You get to nip creativity in the bud.
- You get to teach intolerance.
- You get to start arguments.
- You get to alienate people whom you may need help from later.
- You get to hurt the feelings of the people who love you.
- You get to attract criticism to yourself (out of self-defense.)
- You get to bring disharmony to a peaceful place.
- You get to stifle the dynamics of unity.
- You get to add stress to your life and everyone else's.
- You get to create the conditions for disease. (The most common cause of disease is stress.)
- You get to turn the work place into chaos and discontent.
- You get to stifle artistic creativity.
- You get to invalidate and intimidate others.

- You get to break people's hearts and will.
- You get to break up families.
- You get to make yourself feel that you are better than someone else. Although this is the real payoff, disempowering others to make yourself "right", it doesn't guarantee that they will agree.

Like I've said before, the list is endless. It is a choice. How important is it for us to show how "smart" we are. How smart are we if we are undermining the love, appreciation, praise, and gratitude that make this world a worthwhile place to live? Why make another wrong? What good comes from making someone do something that doesn't agree with their own heart?

We can offer suggestions without criticizing. When someone asks, "Would you like some criticism on (whatever), we cringe. The real answer is , "No!" I want praise. If they say, "What would you think about doing it another way" the listener gets the opportunity to accept the *suggestion* or remain satisfied. Either way, you'll seldom change someone with criticism, but often insult them. But then again, I won't criticize you if you do.

The Colors of Your Life

Before birth we received a life that was empty and meaningless. In a human sense, we are born without opinions, fears, or prejudices. Like an artist's canvas our life is without color, purpose, composition, or meaning. As we grow, we are influenced by people, attitudes, and events. Our *reactions* and the *meanings we add* to the events color our lives. Life itself is neutral. At times our canvas gets splattered with the mud of harsh human experience. This is a good time to step back and observe the appearances and our feelings, so we can recreate our future.

Those who are terrified might cover their canvas with dull grays so that they can blend into the background and avoid confrontation. Others will contrast their life with lights and darks and brilliant colors to give themselves a sense of purpose and self-worth. The latter will, most likely, produce a life of great character and broad appeal. The least desirable option is to decide that life is hard and that people are evil. This mindset serves as an excuse to put away one's creativity and leave the canvas unattended.

If the premise (that life is empty and meaningless) is correct, then it is significant that we were given three gifts at birth: intelligence, intuition, and free will. Having free will, we choose the artist brushes, palettes, and paints with which we color our experience. With these tools in hand, we can paint any scene we wish, from rain clouds to rainbows. There is no limit to the designs, shades, or intensities—the possibilities are limitless. The variables are our beliefs, attitudes, courage, and desires. *Life itself is nothing—but pure potential!*

There is a story of a little boy, curious by nature, who came home from school after his first biology class and asked his mom, "Where did I come from?" The mother, quite embarrassed, summoned her composure and began explaining, in careful detail, the birth process as best she could. After her long, nervous speech, the child exclaimed, "That's cool, Mom! Billy said he came from Pittsburgh."

The other consideration about "meaning" is that everyone has his own. The communication of *facts* can be tricky enough without people adding their own interpretations. We often suffer because of perceptions that were never the intention of the other party. An event occurs. It is what it is—nothing more, nothing less. The meaning added colors it, but doesn't change anything—except the way we have chosen to feel about it. On the other hand, accepting events without judgment or criticism can bring about a feeling of peace and well-being.

Some people spend years trying to "find themselves." They want work befitting their skills that promises higher purpose. Some of these same people hate their jobs and make everyone around them suffer. It seems that they missed the point. If they take a job, no matter what it is, and bring to it enthusiasm, love, integrity, and joy, they are on the path toward their goal. Being on your path adds meaning to jobs, relationships, and life in general. Healthy attitudes attract into people's lives companionship, prosperity, and happiness, which were the real goals anyway. Paint your canvasses accordingly.

Let's remember that *we make the rules*. Our actions and thoughts always have consequences. *Stuff happens*. So what? It always will. Change your thinking and *shift happens!* Get out those brushes and paint your rainbow—and don't forget to paint the pot of gold at the end!

Creating a Better World

"Talent," it has been said, "is created in silence; character, in the stream of life." Let's talk about creating in silence and experiencing higher outcomes in our reality.

A few years back, my dream came true. I had been mentally fishing in my imaginary dream boat for years; now, finally, I bought the real thing. She was shiny and new and had all the contraptions a mariner could wish for to find and catch those rambunctious, silvery, blue-plate specials I enjoy so much. It didn't take more than two or three trips, though, to realize that I had bought a tub. The freeboard was wrong, the floors were slick, and the draft was too deep. I had waited and saved a lifetime (hopefully only half a lifetime) for my ship to come in, and, when it showed up, it was the *Hesperus*.

After sleepless nights and pacing in the gloom, my thinking slowly evolved from what I should have bought to what can I do to create a new, improved dream boat. *What I did next worked so well that I recommend it to anyone who needs a creative solution to any problem.*

First, I sat in silence and stilled my critical mind. In this quieted state I began to write down what I wanted it to be versus what I actually had. I realized that I didn't have a problem, only

42

an unanswered question. I walked past the boat and imagined it looking the way I wanted. In silence my answers came. They seemed radical and illogical, but I made drawings anyway, designing the perfect vessel for my purposes. The process continued for a few days as it evolved.

I don't remember how I found Robby, but after a few phone calls and faxes, I was on a 300-mile journey to have plastic (or should I say fiberglass) surgery performed on my tub.

"Ouch," he gasped, as I showed him the barge. "I didn't know you wanted me to saw a brand new boat in half!" (Horizontally, of course.) However, two weeks later, when I reappeared at his door, his wizardry and my ideas were one. It was a sleek, mean, fishing machine like none other in the world, and at an unbelievably reasonable price! My fishing buddies and I enjoyed many great adventures in my custom craft.

I suspect that others have had similar experiences in problem solving. Even if people are unclear about the benefits of meditation and visualization, when forced to find solutions, many meditate and don't even know that's what they are doing. Meditating can be as simple as quieting the mind, relaxing, trusting, and experiencing mentally what is not seen in the physical world—*yet*. It requires listening and allowing. It is powerful! Proven benefits, by physicians, scientists, and meditators, include better respiration, digestion, and sleep. It can slow aging, reduce stress, focus the mind, aid in healing, and allow answers to appear where none seemed possible. The process allows our intuition to give us a plan. If we write it off as illogical, we usually end up saying, "I knew I should have listened to myself, but whoever dreamed it would turn out this way?"

As Millennium III approaches we can take our creative ability and put it to work, silently meditating and visualizing delightful outcomes for ourselves, our families, friends, country, and planet. We can put our energies on the side of peace and prosperity for Mother Earth, as she has come to be recognized, and her children, the inhabitants. Remember, if we don't *stand* for something now, we will probably *fall* for something later. So join me in meditation, visualization, and expectancy of good. In this way we will surely create a better world.

Integrity

The easiest way to describe integrity is by what it is not. For example, integrity is not lying, cheating, stealing, or in any way harming or depleting others. Integrity includes honor, honesty, sincerity, conviction, wisdom, and other higher human values. *Integrity is the virtue of a person who lives without fear of disapproval*. It means that you would not compromise your highest ideals because you trust these ideals to support you. *Webster's Dictionary* has two definitions of integrity. The first is "courage in character and action." This means that it isn't enough to just speak about or believe in an honorable life style. Commitment and conviction must be proven by deeds of love, honesty, trustworthiness, and courage.

Sometimes integrity is best expressed by standing up to an intimidator or abusive person and letting them know that their behavior will not be tolerated. Most often, however, this is accomplished by merely loving yourself and others too much to accept less than love, truth, and harmony as the standard by which we choose to live.

The second definition is "completeness." Like a structure, if it has integrity (wholeness) it will not collapse under pressure. It is not self-righteousness or indulging ourselves at the cost of others. It is more like empowering ourselves by using our strength to bless others.

Integrity provides the structure and tools to build happiness and prosperity. Character is derived from Love and Principle. These are the cornerstones of all knowledge, growth, business and personal relationships, health, and creative expression.

The next time you feel pressured into compromising your integrity, ask yourself these four questions: (1) What am I afraid of? (2) Do I really want to compromise my health, happiness, or the structure within which I live and hope to spend the rest of my life? (3) Who am I fooling? (4) Do I really believe that the Universe doesn't act under law to give me the fruits of my beliefs, deeds, and actions?

Consider the value and might of your word. If your word doesn't seem powerful, you might want to take a look at your integrity.

Who Am I?

When I was a child my big question was, "Who am I?" After a while I realized that the answers I was getting were all too cynical for this peewee optimist. I still don't have it all figured out, but perhaps you'd like a look at my findings.

The way I see it, it's all about energy. Ask your local physicist and he'll tell you that the matter you call your body is comprised of particles that equate to pluses and minuses or electrical charges. It is energy, he will say, and *energy can be changed but never destroyed*. Our life, our brain, and our planet are a series of electrical impulses manifested as radiation, magnetism, polarity, light, and sound vibrations. The Cosmic and Physical Laws that operate and hold the "material" universe together are gravity, centrifugal force, inertia, adhesion,cohesion, etc. All of these are the result of polarity. Defined in physical terms, polarity is *pure potential*. In metaphysical terms it is *infinite possibility*. What a great substance from which to form a universe! It seems that the metaphysical has finally "come to terms" with the physical.

I hope that this has you all charged up. (Insert apology here for a bad pun.) If you need more facts, consider this: The Russians developed a process whereby they could photograph the energy field surrounding the body. They call it Kirlian photography. This energy field vibrates at a higher rate than the human body and is thereby differentiated. Kirlian photos have shown a hand with a missing finger, albeit the finger's energy field is still intact—sort of like a radiant blueprint of the original. This is proof of the auric body.

So now let's gather the facts. There is a human body comprised primarily of space and electrical impulses. If "particles" were defined as matter, the accumulation of all the matter in a body, minus the empty space, could be condensed to fit on the head of a pin. Further, looking through an electron microscope at the nucleus of an atom, we can see *through* it. Add to this body an auric field that changes colors, size, shape, and intensity according to the mental and emotional energy going on within the individual, and we're only starting to come up with a composite of what we are made of and how we really look.

Let's address the brain, that biological computer that regulates our autonomic nervous system, stores phenomenal amounts of memory, and sorts through it for answers to questions we pose. What an amazing tool! Even the best internationally known physicists can't answer the next question: *Who operates the brain?* Deepak Chopra, author of several books including *Quantum Healing*, says that the question remains unanswered in the field of science. My belief is that I operate my brain, but *Who am I?*

The next time you look in the mirror, instead of counting hairs, pounds, or wrinkles, pause and reflect (what else would you do in a mirror) on who and what you really are. Ask, Am I a mind, existing in what Einstein called the *unified field*, connected to all of the intelligence of the universe, past, present and future? Am I creating my experience by making choices? Am I transporting myself in a wondrous, multicolored, etheric body?

We all are swirling through space, unscathed through planetary mine fields at astronomical speeds, perfectly balanced by physical and spiritual laws. Who I am is *energy*. Who I am eternally is *pure consciousness*. I hope that this knowledge makes you feel energized!

Pulling Yourself Up by Your Bootstraps

I guess we've all had times when life has seemed to be more difficult than we could bear. Disappointments, illnesses, and pressures stacked up endlessly. At such times we may have experienced an "energy failure." If we gave up and went to sleep, we most likely woke up refreshed with new hope and resolve. Amazing how that works.

Renewed energy, after the "letting go" process, results in a new outlook. Sometimes, our subconscious devises a plan while we sleep, and we wake up knowing what to do. When we eventually put together a plan of action, the resolve alone is enough to stop the worry and begin the healing process.

In 1975, while at an all-time low, I turned to my pen and began to write poetry. It was a means of healing then as writing is to me now. The poem, "Freedom's Way," from the Foreword of this book demonstrates how the inspiration that flowed through my pen during this difficult period blessed me.

What a powerful transformation of my spirit! My self-imprisonment was a fear that only love and trust could dispel. How did this inspiration come to me in my darkest hour? I don't really know. Often the flowers of joy come from seeds planted in the soil of despair. So, although I believe in the pot of gold at the end of a rainbow, this doesn't mean I am unaware that rainbows can be preceded by torrential downpours. I'm learning to focus on the spectrum of beautiful possibilities that are inherent in the rainbow while looking forward to the pot of gold (opportunity) that comes as a result of these experiences. The longer and more steadfastly I look for good in the midst of storms, the more frequently I find rainbows on the golden path.

Writing is one way of lifting one's soul. Music is another. Dancing, singing, or playing a musical instrument are all methods of releasing sadness and attuning oneself to the rhythm of life. Arts and crafts likewise bring out our personal creativity. Games like tennis, golf, or bridge can enable us to return to our childlike playfulness. In such a state we are freed from self-imposed worries.

Sadness is usually attributable to either worry, guilt, or grief. *Grief* is a feeling of deep personal loss. Patience with oneself, gratitude for that which is good in one's life, forgiveness, and a desire to move out of the pain is the recommended remedy. Laughter and the sharing of love and joy with others can also regenerate the soul.

It is OK to overcome *guilt* instantly because time spent feeling guilty is time wasted. Have no reverence for guilt. It should not be mistaken for earnest concern. It is punishing and destructive to the spirit. Without criticism or self-criticism, guilt doesn't exist.

Worry is a sickness that drains our energy. It is an immobilizing fear of what *might* happen. That which we worry about rarely occurs. When that which we feared actually happens, we can handle it—especially if we don't flow our energy to issues that aren't real. When we waste energy, flowing it where it blesses no one, *it comes right out of our health centers. Choose wisely how you flow your Life Force!*

If pulling yourself up by the bootstraps is the order of your day, know that you can do it. You have every mechanism needed to enjoy a healthy, happy life. Use these tools we've discussed and rediscover the joy that is your birthright.

The Secret Behind Charisma

We all know someone who is so special that we call them charismatic. Chances are, as you read that sentence, someone came to mind—a person who is always "up," who has amazing energy, whose touch turns straw into gold. This special one is calm, yet exciting; loving, but not demanding nor dependent; interested, but not nosy; multitalented, but focused on the business at hand; successful, but not arrogant. A balanced person such as this has problems like you and I but doesn't express them as complaints. To these people trials are stepping stones along the path to the fulfillment of their dreams.

What makes the charismatic person special? Common sense? Maybe, although there is nothing common about it. Love? Very much so, but not in an emotional, external way. Commitment? In part. Wishy, washy just doesn't cut it.

"Well, why is it," you ask, "that we admire these people so much?"

I believe that it is their zeal for life. In a word, *enthusiasm*. The word enthusiasm has its root in the Greek *theos* meaning God. To be infused with the spirit of God would surely explain the empowerment of those focused on and excited about their life and purpose.

To be enthusiastic is to expect good and relish each small event as it occurs. Enthusiasm is love for Life, for nature, and for things man-made. For sunshine, children at play, friends, new discoveries, giving, receiving, and the multitude of blessings we would otherwise tend to take for granted in our everyday lives. In short, what makes certain people attract us is their *chosen* ability to hold as precious each glorious day with every-one and everything in it. The attitude that says, "Today is wondrous and I don't want to miss a moment of it" or "You're special and I appreciate you" or "I can't wait to see how Life will unfold for me today!" The attitude that says, "Everyone and everything I see is how the Universe is ex-pressing through me—what a joy it is to be alive!"

William James, known as the father of functional psychology, said that feeling *follows* action. Dale Carnegie took this principle to his classrooms and taught, "Act enthusiastic and you'll be enthusiastic" to thousands who proved its efficacy by bringing success into their lives. If Charles Fillmore, co-founder of Unity, could say, "I fairly sizzle with enthusiasm ..." at the age of 94, so can you and I!

Let's not focus upon the petty negatives that present themselves daily; instead, reject them in favor of gratitude for the millions of things that go right every day. Let's lavish praise upon those who so seldom hear the words of encour-agement they deserve, and let's get fired up about the power of good in our lives. These steps will evoke the Universal Law of Attraction that brings to us that which we contemplate. Therefore, consider enthusiasm. It is the jump-starter. It is that which we can bring to any situation to start the flow of good. It is how we can attract what we want into our experience. It is the irresistible energy of Life expressing through us! It is love in action! It is the secret behind Charisma.

Making Coincidences Work for You

When I took Science of Mind classes, we studied the works of many fine authors: Emerson, Troward, and Ernest Holmes included. What they teach in common with today's motivational speakers is that our words, beliefs, and thoughts dramatically affect our lives. In our classes and the writers' texts, we learned of the power of affirmations. I practiced the concepts. In my mind, it was an exercise about instilling new habits using self-talk. After all, could the words you speak, perhaps only once, magically change your life experience? How specific could the process really be? My question was soon to be answered.

When I bought my nifty little fishing rig, I hoped it would improve my lot as a fisherman. My recent trips had been, to say the least, a little boring. I affirmed with conviction, *"I have exciting fishing trips!"* On the next two fishing trips my boat was nearly swamped, and my friend and I had to fend for our lives. I got the message. I realized how specific I would need to be when programing my mind in the future. I changed my affirmation to *"I have wonderful, safe, and productive fishing trips."* Since then, not only have I learned to avoid or deal with the problems that previously endangered me, but my trips have been blessed with visits from dolphins, manatees, ospreys, and other beautiful wildlife.

Telling stories like this has caused me to leave a wake of skepticism through the years. In the past, I have had the joyful little miracles that have followed my study, prayer, affirmations, visualizations, and Reiki energy work deemed *coincidences* by many; I have been considered radical by others. Nevertheless, making "coincidences" work for me has become a way of life.

Today, there is less resistance to this philosophy than ever before. When I was six years old and spoke of the power of the mind imbued with spiritual intent, my school teachers felt accosted. I used biblical scripture to make my point. This was embarrassing for them as they didn't know scripture well enough to argue with me. As a child, I was quite zealous. Since then, I have learned to temper my tongue—a little. *I don't push a religion, nor do I subscribe to any philosophy that says "I am right and you are wrong."* My philosophy is nondenominational and says that I am right for me—until I make a mistake. Then I revise my philosophy, correct the mistake if possible, and keep learning new ways to live my life better. My belief is this: "You are right for you and I have no right to try to change you." If, however, anything I say, do, or write resonates with you and you can use it, then I get the added benefit of sharing myself—and that feels good.

Affirmations and sound self-talk are quick and easy ways to begin the journey of using our own mind to change our life. If we add desire and/or belief, we empower the process. If we see, in our mind's eye, the finished result of our desire, we become a visionary. Our dreams are not necessarily whimsical. They can be powerful tools. We need not let our logical mind (or another's) talk us out of our power to create. By believing in ourselves and putting into words an affirmation, we have taken the first step toward making it a reality.

There is nothing that we own that wasn't first an idea, and secondly a spoken word. Those things we have not manifested remain devoid of clear thought and conscious declaration. It is not likely to create something without devotion of thought and desire. Possibilities, however, are limitless...and so are we!

The Commuter

I'd like to relate a story told to me back in 1964 by my late teacher, Grace V. Dickinson, C.S.B.

There was an elderly lady in New York, who daily took the bus to work. Each morning she would climb into the bus, pay her fare, and say "Good morning" to the driver. He would ignore her and never return her greeting.

On one such morning, she got on the bus, paid her fare, said "Good morning," and went back and sat down. The lady seated next to her commented, "Every morning for months now I have watched you pleasantly greet that grouchy bus driver, and every day he totally ignores you. Why do you bother?"

The little lady replied with a knowing smile, "I'm not going to let *his behavior* change what I am!"

Don't you just love her conviction? *We all need to know the inner part of us where our highest ideals identify us*, where the light of love pierces the fog of human fears and frustrations. It happens in the lives of every one of us. Unfortunately, we usually hurry back to the illusion of fear and confusion that we call "reality" and put our ideal aside *as though our intrinsic wisdom and power were the temporary sense of things.* It doesn't have to be that way.

Each day we see the best and the worst in everyone. At times like this we come face to face with our real Self and compare it to our counterfeit self. Unfortunately, we are far too hard on ourselves. We can think that a mistake we made in the past proves that we are basically unlovable today. We don't remember the child, born of perfect love, that resides in our heart. When afraid of making changes, we say, "I guess that's just the way I am" with a "take it or leave it" attitude, as though a behavior could be etched in stone for eternity.

We are evolving. We are not static. Anything is possible. It is less painful to choose change and growth than to ignore our evolution. We seem to have bought into unnecessary pressures, burning the candle at both ends. It is better to listen to the inner voice and slow down than to keep running until we "hit the wall."

When we are rushing around, we fly through life without dealing with the issues that require quiet contemplation. We need to look at ourselves deeply so that we may find the beauty within that will make us feel good about ourselves once more. We can exchange our previous fear-motivated behavior for the deep joy of forgiveness and compassion. Let's seize the opportunity and let light and love shine through us. Let us not forget who we *really* are!

Making Tough Decisions

Usually, when a tough decision comes up we like to bounce our options off someone we believe has our best interests at heart. This is usually helpful because we need to express clearly what we are thinking. Probably, this person is not lost in the same "forest" as we are and can see the situation more clearly.

Ever have someone ask your opinion and, as soon as you make your choice, they pick the opposite? This is how the sounding board approach works. They weren't sure what they wanted until they felt their response to your choice.

There are some yes/no choices that are easy because of the Law of Cause and Effect, which promises us a consequence to deal with for every thought and action. For most decisions, we are well qualified intellectually. Often we like to procrastinate, hoping that no choice will be necessary. Beware of the Law of Default, which states that if you choose not to choose, the result will be random, probably not to your liking, and will interfere with your self-empowerment process and future plans.

My dad used to say to me, "Confidence is built by a series of successful experiments." Take pride in the ninety-five percent of your decisions that come easily based upon your love, awareness, intuitiveness, good logic, experience, and integrity. You will find that most of these decisions, even if made incorrectly, can easily be corrected or improved upon. After all, who do you know with a perfect record? Trust that even if your action brings an unwelcome outcome, the Universe will always support you in that which you must do to make adjustments and get on with your life.

We can become aware of our fears and motivations to see what is driving us in any direction, and quiet the confused, critical mind in deference to the intuitive part of us that already knows what is best. Recoiling in fear is a mistake. Going forward in trust with an open mind is far better. In a state of stillness we can proceed with the absolute conviction that there is always a good answer. In fact, there are many good answers if we can let go of our past-based thinking.

We get impressions and feelings that guide us. Intuition, a sense to be reckoned with, can come as an inner knowing that often has no logic to support it. It can be scary to act on something when you don't know how you know it! If you don't act on it you'll probably say later, "Why didn't I listen to myself?" Neither fear, imaginings, doubt, nor discouragement should be allowed to stifle our creative flow.

Some powerful techniques taught in MIT-trained Pete A. Sanders, Jr.'s book, *You Are Psychic*, include (a) focusing on your solar plexus (gut area) to see how your answers *feel*,

(b) closing your eyes to *see* where your thoughts are leading you, (c) listening to hear the voice *within*, or (d) just allowing yourself to have an *instant knowing* that can reveal your path. You are naturally powerful in *at least* one of these four areas. These techniques can help you find where *you* best access *your* higher information. Answers will unfold at the most amazing times and under the strangest conditions. Practice until you learn to trust your inner Self.

In truth, there are no coincidences, no mistakes, and no failures to the person focused on love and integrity, who moves forward without being judgmental, and who is motivated to bless others. In my life, my errors have taught me that I am the creator of my experiences; that I alone make myself happy or sad and, most importantly, that the Universe always supports me in the achievement of an honest goal.

I leave you with this challenge: Having only an instant to make a momentous decision, I'd blow logic to the wind and go with my gut every time. What about you?

Shaping Our Destiny

We may not always be aware, but we are the designers and architects of our own lives. While we might give credit or blame to others, in reality, it is not what happens to us or around us that shapes our destiny, as much as it is what we do with these circumstances.

Our vision takes us from where we are to where we are going. Only our fears and doubts can block our progress in the long run. Doubts are limiting beliefs and feelings. They say, "I can't handle it" or "I'd better not try" or "Maybe someone more qualified than me..."

We are the ones in our lives who make the choices. We choose the building materials (what we eat and drink). We choose whether or not we smoke or use drugs. This brings to mind a story about my recently departed aunt. She was remembering how she started smoking. She, a nonsmoker, married Charlie, a smoker. He insisted that she try it—just to be sociable. She did and became a heavy smoker for the next half-century. Here she was in her seventies before she realized that it was never her idea in the first place. My aunt became furious at herself and her long ago deceased ex-husband and quit smoking then and there. Was she a victim? Yes—*a victim of her own choices.* Charlie only made a suggestion, nothing more. He was powerless in her life until she bought his idea. We err in blaming others for our mistakes, thereby giving away our power.

When confronting a situation we can take steps to quiet doubt, make better choices, affirm our good, and refocus our attention on a higher purpose. We must have a vision if we would design a more beautiful and purposeful life. We can't hit the mark if we don't have a target. If we lift our sights, we can design a much richer, happier life.

"Feeling Good"

So much of the time we feel like we are carrying the weight of the world on our shoulders. Many years ago, a caring friend, noting my tendency to carry the burdens of others, teasingly suggested that I resign my self-appointed job as *General Manager of the Universe.* This shocking remark forced me to realize that my self-inflicted pressure was unnecessary, energy draining, and worse, nobody was going to appreciate it. False responsibility is not caring—it is meddling!

Why is it so hard to *feel good* all of the time? Looking back, there must have been ten thousand times when I thought that I was in a serious situation. Buying into the temporary conditions that appeared in my life extended their stay. Clearly recognizing that they are subject to a change of consciousness made a huge difference in my life. *A change of attitude always creates a change in one's experience.*

Remember, *ninety percent of everything that we worry about never occurs!* As explained earlier in this book, this liberating truth implies that we can handle the ten percent more easily if we disregard the unnecessary ninety percent. I usually can't even remember those things that had me hammered with anxiety two weeks ago.

Having survived for decades, I can surmise that it is within my scope to *feel good* about today.

Just before she passed away, my mother-in-law gifted me. We were all at her bedside. She lay there unconscious, not having uttered a word all day. Knowing that she was a devout Catholic, when the family left the room for food, I went to her side to speak words that I believed would make her *feel well*. Not knowing how it would impact the situation, I whispered, "God loves you." Suddenly, her eyes flashed open and she began speaking, rapidly recounting many events from her life. She chuckled about the dogs, grandchildren, her family, on and on. She repeated six life-changing words three times, *"Never, never be afraid of anything."* There, on what people would call her death bed, she was telling me not to be afraid—of anything!

Pause and visualize yourself traveling into outer space for a moment, and look back at our tiny, blue, water planet. Considering the big picture, what is really important? Isn't it about *being happy and letting others around us catch this infectious delight?* Why let fear, doubt, worry, and pressure of time deprive us of our innate joy? Wanna *feel good*? Sing a happy tune. How would you feel if you danced in front of your mirror singing "I'm So Excited" or "Celebrate" or "*I Feel Good*"? Try it, it's dynamite!

Let me also suggest this: If you feel happy singing, dancing, painting, biking, swimming, or whatever, do it more! If someone says that you have to do something that doesn't resonate with you, ask "Who made these rules?" If they are not sound, *make new rules that bring you joy. Keep on feeling good and spreading that feeling!*

Finding Our Treasures

Ever remember being down and out? When nothing goes our way, we start believing that it never will. That's OK, for a while. Leaving reality to visit the fantasy world of "If I Buy Something I Will Feel Better" enables us to temporarily ignore our unresolved issues. However, when we go back home, the problems are still waiting for us, and so are the additional bills. Neither our money nor our possessions bring consolation at a time like this.

Money is good for a multitude of purposes. I spend a great deal of time figuring out how I can exchange services for money. Even so, money is being rapidly replaced by plastic and will soon be given a back seat by computer-driven shopping systems. Money, in one form or another, is part of our life plans and these plans represent to many of us a joy in life. Having a plan and pursuing it gives us a renewed sense of self-worth and excitement. Money is the middle part, not the start nor end of the process. Our dreams initiate our plans and our choices determine the outcome.

Did you ever know anyone who wanted any *thing*, then somehow got it and was thereafter satisfied for the rest of their life? Life is an ongoing process. We never really "arrive," we just keep traveling. Everything in our life requires maintenance. Whether it is replacing light bulbs and dusting a lamp or bringing home the puppy so that we can feed, groom, and scoop poop in all kinds of weather for the next eighteen years, if we want something, we are required to care for it.

Our greatest gift, in my estimation, is our mind. We use it to direct our lives. But how do we treat it? We can nourish it with life-enhancing information and gentle meditation or we can fill it with trash: gossip, complaint, and criticism. Affirmations of love and Universal support for a few moments each day can do more to free our minds to better serve us than weeks or months of conniving how to get our fingers on something that we will tire of quickly.

Our second greatest gift is our body. Although not every body fits the mold of Mr. or Miss America, it is, nevertheless, our priceless tool box. A facial expression can tell a story that the spoken or written language can only hope to mimic. Our hands, feet, nervous system, and senses serve us well so that we can detect and respond with appropriate choices that will enhance our quality of life. Ask someone who is missing one of these great gifts, and they will tell you how valuable each and every part and system of the body is. What can we do to care for this otherwise self-maintaining body? Overloading its vascular, endocrine, and digestive systems with "food" that is so unnatural that there is no way it ever belonged inside a human is not the way.

Instead, we can properly feed and exercise this tool so that its systems will thrive.

Another major gift is our environment. We can help keep our environment clean and safe by enjoying nature without abusing it. We can do our part, and hopefully just a little extra, to prevent further accumulation of toxicity by working for and demanding clean soil, air, and water. We need to protect and care for our planet and resources.

Finally, when shopping and TV fail to console our lonely hearts, there is the gift of *friendship*. Whether it be a spouse, relative, business associate, or just a pal who listens, life takes on a new meaning when we share our feelings, dreams, and even our plights with a caring friend. Gratitude and genuine appreciation serve best in maintaining friendships. What treasures are our friends! Choose well; these are the chief ingredients in a happy and successful life.

There are those who would confront me: "Don't try telling me that money is just a *state of mind* because I won't buy it! (oops a bad pun...) You've said that health can be determined by one's attitudes and beliefs and maybe I can see a relationship between how we feel psychologically and physiologically. You've said that our attitudes attract people in or out of our lives. There might be some truth to that, but *bucks are bucks* and what has attitude got to do with money?"

Dollars are merely a means of exchange. They are neutral, powerless, meaningless. *We* give them their power and meaning. If we give them the power in our lives to make or break us, then and only then can they master us. Our attitudes about money are much more important than the money itself. We all know happy people who have little money and wealthy people who are miserable. There are ex-millionaires who are now bankrupt and underprivileged people who have made it to the top. Some people have a surplus of money and are happy, but that is much harder to do, because we, as a nation, seem to be insatiable. Nothing ever seems to be enough. Each time we see a few extra bucks, we take a trip or buy something we want (but probably don't need). This is fine *IF* we don't complain after we've spent the money that we're broke again. Without the complaint, the process of getting money and spending it is basically acceptable.

As if insatiability isn't self-defeating enough, there are many of us who can't even wait until we have a few dollars to spend them. We borrow (usually against credit cards) and spend it without even having earned it. Is this not a perfect example of a *state of mind* that keeps us from prospering? If we are paying a credit card company fifteen to eighteen percent interest on vacations that are long behind us, how are we to get ahead?

The question, therefore, is not, "How much money do I need to be happy?" That never ends. It is more like, "How much delight can I find in my life with what I have now?"

Prosperous thinking and honest service attract money. *The only way to be happy is to decide to be happy—and that, my dear, dear friend, is a state of mind!*

Up in Flames

Flames suddenly appeared, drawing my undivided attention. The hibachi chef cut, diced, and juggled our dinners with the point of his razor-sharp knife. He then twirled his blade and slid it into its holster like a western gunslinger.

As I applauded his dexterity and culinary skills, it was evident that I was the only one child-like enough to appreciate the show. I sounded like the lone clapper at the end of a "Laugh In" episode. The other nine people sat silently, watching their dinner cooking, impatiently awaiting its completion.

Their blasé attitude painfully reminded me of how we seem to be evolving into a "quick-fix" society. As a group, we need constant amusement. We are in such a rush to go nowhere. If there is a lull, we whip out our credit card or cellular phone to make something happen. Our relationships, health, and finances are in disrepair from neglect; meanwhile, we pop aspirins and stomach acid pills so that we can rush through another cheeseburger on the way to the department stores or movie theater. Our bodies nag us for nourishment, so we placate them with caffeine or alcohol. Our children and mates beg us to share our lives, so we make promises that we can't deliver, and then get angry when we are reminded. Is this prosperity? As a massage therapist and Reiki master, I observe, with amazement, the stress that people carry in their minds and bodies, with no plan whatsoever to release it!

Optionally, I prefer to take an occasional weekend off to do things like calling old friends or meditating on the direction of my life. Can you remember the last time you took your significant other to a park to hold hands and walk side by side? Here in Florida we have the most beautiful skies. I love to watch a gorgeous sunset and then spend an evening on the beach star-gazing.

Possessions can distract our attention from who and what we are. Tools and comforts are great, but *if we pay more attention to our "things" than our spiritual and emotional needs, we feel distress.* Clutter and incomplete tasks nag at us until we deal with them.

It is always a good time to pause and take a serious look at how we are dispersing our energies. If we are not peaceful and grateful, we might decide to give up activities that don't serve our health and happiness. We can care for our own physical, emotional, and spiritual needs. We can improve our eating habits and exercise properly. We can do little kindnesses for friends and strangers. We can work on our completeness so that we are not dependent on others more than necessary. We can take time to be grateful for the host of benefits that life offers. We can read positive materials to be reminded that we are truly blessed.

It was May of 1997, and I was at a Carolyn Myss seminar in Orlando. Ms. Myss had spent some time showing us how energy flows through our bodies, minds, and experience. She then asked a member of the audience to tell her what percentage of her energy she expended in maintaining her personal relationships, then her work, then her home upkeep, and so on. When totaled, she had enumerated about one hundred and fifty percent! We laughed, but Ms. Myss did not. She drove home the point that if we wake up in the morning with one hundred and fifty percent of our energy already committed, we are building up an energy debt. This energy deficiency must come from our bodies at a deep cellular level. To pay this debt would insure illness.

She admonished us, "Be careful where and how you flow your energy."

How do you feel when you pass a messy room? Or a pile of unpaid bills? What happens to your heart when the name of a person with whom you have unfinished issues comes up? What happens in the pit of your stomach when you believe you have harmed someone? Remember, a change in your thinking can instantly create a change in your energy. How do you feel when someone appreciates the job you've done well? What do you feel when someone remembers an act of kindness that you once committed? How does it feel when you finally get the garage cleaned? When you hold your child or grandchild? When you're sitting at the end of the day and your cat curls up in your lap or when Rover sits at your feet? What happens to your energy at times like these?

There are energizers such as sharing love, gratitude, enthusiasm, laughter, appreciation, accomplishment, giving, receiving, playing, and listening to our favorite music. On the other hand, fear, resentment, undisciplined waste of time, criticism, complaint, and judgmentalism are drains on the soul. They leave us with no rewards, only a false sense of control. The consciousness that blesses is continually energized.

Let us not, however, leave this message unbalanced. Being benevolent doesn't mean that the giver has no needs. Just as the tide must come in before it can go out, we must take our joy and spiritual nourishment from life before we can give of ourselves. Resting is not the same as being lazy. Giving away that which we need for our own well-being is poor budgeting, not generosity. The balancing of our energies is vital to our health and benefits those who depend upon us.

We are never depleted by giving love. We can, however, be depleted by giving away our lives to others because we doubt our own worth. Watch carefully how you flow your energy. Let joy, enthusiasm, and gratitude flow from your heart and you will always have an abundance of life force energy!

Our Ministry

A while ago my brother told me that his work left him feeling empty. He wanted his life to have meaning, but where was he to find "spiritual work?" I remembered Marianne Williamson's words on her "Course in Miracles" tape. She said that "anyone with an address book has a ministry." I added that we are all here to "minister" to each other, that is, to care for one another.

"It is not necessary for you or me to save the world single-handedly," I explained. "We can help and heal anyone we meet anytime, any place." We don't need our own church or environmental agency to take our stand in life. *The intention of our conscious thought is powerful and outreaching beyond our wildest dreams*. Who we are and how we live is our sermon. Whom we meet, and with whom we speak, determines our congregation. Regardless of our profession, there are people who interact with us. If we give them a smile, validate their feelings, or just show some appreciation, we can heal their hearts. If our example points to a higher way of life, we are healers and teachers.

Then I told him the beliefs that I wish to embody and share. One might call them "My Ministry"...

- *Be grateful. The shortcut to all happiness is gratitude.*
- *It is not what happens to us that counts, it is how we respond.*
- *See the best in everyone. You can't be better than that which you see in other people.*
- *Embrace life, it is miraculous.*
- *Focus on the ninety percent that is going right in your world and trust your spiritual intuition with the other ten percent.*
- *If you want to change the world—replace complaint, criticism, and judgmentalism with love and appreciation.*
- *Replace the three most useless emotions—worry, guilt, and doubt—with love, appreciation, and trust.*

Why not write down the message you want to share with the world. Let that be your sermon and deliver it, BY YOUR EXAMPLE.

The Mystical Secrets of Life

It hit me like a ton of bricks. One by one the pieces came together. How foolishly I was pursuing the secrets of life!

From early childhood I was asking, "Why am I here? What is my purpose? Why was I born?"

A few years ago, while contemplating my disappointments, I drifted back about thirty years to my teenage aspirations. They were a wife, a small house, a car, a job where I could excel, peace, and happiness. I imagined how I would have felt if, back then, I could have looked into a crystal ball and seen my life as it is now.

"Wow!" I thought. "Who'd ever dream that I would own a ranch-style home in Florida." (Back in New Jersey, where I was raised, houses were old, multilevel, multifamily dwellings with tiny dark rooms, radiators, pigs feet bathtubs, and dingy basements—ranches were for richer people.)

The list continues: an office in my home where I could write and hold healing sessions for friends and acquaintances. My teenage eyes scanned my middle-age possessions, including my sporty Nissan. Foreign cars, in the sixties, were rare and indicated status. Computers, TV sets with VCRs, stereos with CD players, and best of all, a fishing boat.

"Neat!" I would have said. Certainly my modest possessions today would be a marvel to a teenager back in the sixties. Nevertheless, I realized that I had exceeded all of my expectations in life. Truly, all my dreams came true—and more!

Obviously, comparisons are a source of discontent. This was a powerful awakening. Like so many other people I know, I was beating myself up for my imagined failures. Contemplation of this has since led me to the following perceptions:

- *The greatest of secrets are merely the smallest of virtues.*
- *These virtues exist within all of us.*
- *Seeking them outside of ourselves is foolishness.*

Consider the following "Acres of Diamonds" true story, which I believe I heard during a Dale Carnegie Seminar. In short, a man sold his farm to go out in pursuit of riches. He spent the rest of his life searching for a diamond mine. He died sick and penniless. The farm he sold turned out to be located on what became the largest diamond mine in history. This is the story of you and me! Our greatness or richness is not *out there* somewhere—it is here, within each one of us.

Balance (being centered), to me, is one of the great secrets in life. It means avoiding extreme, radical, or combative thinking. Imagine how much greater this country would be if political parties would stop fighting and instead expend

81

all of their energy working together for the good of us all! Unbalanced (eccentric) thinking in our personal life affects our health and relationships similarly. When our thinking is balanced, our choices are clearer, our objectives are plain, and our actions are more decisive. If we spent more time in quiet contemplation, we would spend less time correcting mistakes. If we take the time to quietly create peace in our lives each day, we will marvel at how much more we can accomplish— with energy left over!

I recently spoke on the telephone to a friend I had lost touch with thirty years ago. I told her how I joyfully remembered her bright eyes and warm smile like it was yesterday. I could hear the tears in her voice as she thanked me for remembering the person she really was, and not letting the years mottle my vision. It touched my heart to be able to share this moment with her. Joy cannot exist in any other mental climate except love.

Occasionally coming face to face with love, yields *part-time* joy. Let's not motivate our lives by fear. Instead of making choices from the persuasion of past experience, we can choose from the possibilities that exist in the future where options are limitless. Live love, and...live life enthusiastically!

Your Ideal Mate

But what of romance? It brings joy to our hearts to see lovers walking hand in hand, smiling dreamily. Like watching an angelic child sleeping, it is a reminder of the most tender moments in life that seem to touch us on the deepest level. When we see them, we feel the glow of our own fond memories.

Sometimes, however, we hold concern over the storms that will test the love of this, perhaps unsuspecting, happy couple. We remember the hardships of past love relationships—the struggles from money management difficulties, or disappointments when romance faded and routine set in, or worse, the pain of crushed dreams when we watched the "love of our life" walk out the door. Although these events shaped our character, nevertheless it can feel sad to remember.

Yet love in its eternal nature lives on and another day dawns with new hopes, dreams, and a myriad of possibilities. We watch as millions of hopeless romantics dream of that perfect other who will change their inadequate lives into a perfect dream world.

"Wait!" you say, "no one wants to be 'hopeless,' and we can't create good relationships by dreaming that someone else will make us whole."

True, no one out there is going to make us happy if we are not inclined to be happy. All we have to do is listen to couples bickering to know that people who look to someone else for their happiness are miserable. *If I can't be everything that I want to be,* how can I expect that of my mate? Wouldn't she want to be appreciated for being her own wonderful, evolving self? She certainly doesn't want to be some stereotype I invented and am trying to mold her into—a stereotype that I don't plan to change myself to fit.

Great relationships come from people appreciating each other in spite of their differences, not from two people with low self-esteem sticking together in hope of becoming one whole person.

And what is true love? It is healthy, loving people coming together to share who and what they are, openly and honestly. True love is seeing the good in our partner and encouraging it. It is seeing areas of conflict and implementing compromise for the sake of continuance. It is doing little things to remind our loved one of how precious he or she is. It is patience in adversity. It is caring for each other, but not inflicting our will on our partner. It is mutual trust and respect. It is a safe place for sharing our successes and our disappointments.

Healthy relationships are not just about getting our needs met, nor being expected to meet someone else's needs. *It is being there for each other while each learns to meet his or her own needs*. True love brings happiness when we find someone to *share* our dreams, not to *fill* them. Romance is a lovely, fleeting fantasy. True love grows because it is nurtured by both parties.

Romantic love can be full of emotion and impossible expectations. It can sweep us off our feet (and out of our minds). When lovers drop each other cues and say the words that their beloved longs to hear, the mating ritual begins. The follow up is wooing (the sales job), entertaining each other, dreaming, and making plans. It can be a very happy time as most everyone wants to be loved and many enjoy making another happy.

After awhile though, someone realizes that there are compromises or, even worse, inconveniences being introduced into the partnership. It is at this critical point that many relationships hit the rocks. This is good news. If someone will leave because of an inconvenience, it is better not to embark into a life with that person.

If the two survive hard times without bruising each other, there is a possibility of a real friendship in the offing. If there is *mutual respect* and genuine *mutual support*, the ingredients are present for a loving relationship with many possibilities. Without these two aspects in place, in my estimation, there is no reason whatsoever for the two to be together. Marriages or arrangements where either or both nag, insult, belittle, criticize, or demoralize one another most of the time are ill-fated. Yet many people choose to live like that because they are afraid to be alone.

My brother once told me, "You teach people how to treat you." Consider this when criticizing another's behavior.

Another problem that can occur is "unreasonable expectations." Many want their mate to be perfect. They believe that their mate should complement them in all possible areas. This need probably arises out of a feeling of inadequacy. When people feel good about themselves they can live with their beloved regardless of differences, enjoying their loving and supportive company when together and being able to occupy themselves happily with their own activities when their mate is elsewhere. Our mate is someone with whom to share time and space, love and memories. We don't own any other person.

It is good when couples work together for the common good with a minimum of grumbling, a maximum of enthusiasm for life, and a sincere desire for the happiness of the other—*but not at the cost of their own identity or self-respect*. It does sound like a lot to balance, but it is you who makes the choices that make your life joyful or dreary. You choose your activities, your attitudes about them, the people in your lives, how you treat them, and how you allow them to treat you.

Check out the following questions about relationships. Can you answer "yes" to all of these questions?

- Do you respect your mate?
- Are you supportive of your mate?
- Do you love and respect yourself?
- Do you speak kindly of each other when you are apart?
- Do you smile inside when you hear your mate's name or voice?

If the answers are "yes," then rejoice in your good fortune. If there are areas that are vague or negative, then it is time to make new choices of some sort. We can support our mate by giving encouragement. We can empower ourselves in areas of self-esteem. If we have a problem that doesn't easily respond to our efforts and our love life doesn't work, then perhaps it is time to find a good counselor to put things in perspective. My belief is this: "We can't do *nothing*." We are the ones who can change our lives.

If the love relationship seems to be acceptable, we must keep working at it anyway. Ignore it and it could go away. We can decide to rebuild it anew. Our choice can be to say, "I love myself and therefore I can love you." Anything less and everyone is being cheated. To receive respect we must give respect. If we want someone to love us, we must love ourselves. To find the right person, *be* the right person.

There is no substitute for a commitment to love. The key is mutuality. If we would keep our loved one, it might be a good idea to get together and *each write out an agreement of mutual promises and expectations*. A lot can be learned if both parties are truthful. This could be observed well before an intended marriage or partnership of any kind. The partners could rehearse every possible problem in their minds and decide if they really could coexist with the conditions. In spite of all the talk about unconditional love, relationships are very conditional. Love is, by definition, unconditional. Anything else is not love; it is a relationship, a mutual agreement, an insecurity or yearning. *Only unconditional love is love*.

First and foremost, the most important condition for a lasting relationship is mutual respect, the second is real friendship, the third is trust, and finally a deep love and appreciation. By this I mean caring, not romance. Romance can be preserved, but without these elements it cannot endure the blasts of time and experience.

The extra advantage to the agreement is that it can be used on each anniversary as a renewal vow. Of course, if both parties wish to improve the agreement and mutually make changes as they grow together, they can. It enables the understanding to continue and reminds the partners of the dedication they had from the beginning.

Let not fear be the motive in picking one's mate. None of us is perfected yet, but we can be working towards emotional health. Growing together is part of the joy of relationships. Your ideal mate can only show up for you when you are open, willing, and self-fulfilled. If you're waiting for someone to cure your ills, see a professional. If you want a partner, be a whole person and choose a whole person. *Be a beacon of light, and then rest assured that your ship will come in.*

"Unless it's mad, passionate, extraordinary love, it is a waste of your time. There are too many mediocre things in life; love shouldn't be one of them."

—from "Dreams for an Insomniac"

What Is This World Coming To?

Only 150 years ago, in order to survive in this country it was necessary, at a moment's notice, to be prepared to fend for your life. Times were barbaric, and the land was wild and treacherous. Life expectancy was short, and living conditions were hard. The probability of surviving a cross-country journey by wagon train was poor. Forging rivers, climbing mountains, blazing trails, extreme weather, circumnavigating obstacles, and battling hostile gangs or tribes was a normal part of life. Thus was the history of man from the beginning of recorded time until later in the nineteenth century, when changes began to accelerate.

Today, millions travel daily without fear of a marauding tribe or gang coming to rob and destroy their little "caravan" or burn and kill their families. Whew! Things really are a lot better than we have been realizing, aren't they? Of course, some people still choose to live in fear of such possibilities despite the fact that life, in general, is not that way any more. Perhaps this is due to the cellular memory of millions of years of human history handed down and stored in our DNA. Perhaps certain people's paranoia is based on the fact that they are situated in a place (they haven't yet chosen to leave) that *actually is* an isolated pocket of modern-day barbarism. Regardless of why this state of consciousness persists, now is a great time to open our eyes to the overwhelming good that is taking over our world.

I believe that this transition began in the mid-nineteenth century with great thinkers such as Ralph Waldo Emerson, Phineas T. Quimby, Mary Baker Eddy, Emma Curtis Hopkins, and others who taught and proved that spirituality is a mental *science* with limitless possibilities that is available to everyone. As a result of the efforts of these and other visionaries, we find ourselves facing the greatest period of accelerated understanding since recorded time on our young dynamic planet–welcome, Millennium III –we're ready!

What is this world coming to? Never before have there been so many groups and individuals banding together for the care and preservation of people in need, animals, and our enviroment. It is no longer necessary to hide behind an obsolete "we vs. them" defensive attitude. We can choose to desire the best for everyone because it is becoming so very obvious that we live in a limitless universe and that another's success doesn't necessitate our lack.

Possibilities abound! Anyone can have anything that he or she can concieve and believe in. The proof is in the unwritten biographies of those millions of unsung heroes/heroines who have braved unbelievable odds in their anonymous lives, and have reached heights attainable only by those who are willing to subject their fears and doubts to their dream and desires. Their successes were due to their ability to replace the temptation of self-pity and doubt with courage, acceptance, and vision.

We have the ability and opportunity to empower our fellow man, nurture our planet, and advance ourselves as never before. It is time to lift our thinking beyond the 11:00 news reports and soap operas—real or televised—and turn the aspirations of science fiction into reality. We can be part of that mentality that lifts world consciousness. Today, many have already begun to pursue this pathway. Tomorrow we will be remembered as those who had the vision to change the world. Let's share our commitment to this higher standard.

What's this world coming to? *The heights of mental and spiritual power*. How is it manifesting? *As human love and caring—as commitment to the very highest ideals*. Let us lead the way to making the world a better place by raising consciousness through expectancy, visualization, and service to mankind.

The Reality Check

OK, so you're out diving and find an oyster. (a) You might open the oyster, take the pearl, and chuck the remains into the sea. Sound right so far? Now try this. (b) You're stranded on a desert island. You dive in the water and find an oyster. You break open the nasty little bivalve, suck down the creature, careful to throw away the pearl before it gets caught in your throat. Who needs a pearl when there is no one around but you and survival is the only order of the day? (c) While swimming underwater, you observe an oyster, but have too much respect for life to ever touch the little creature for fear of harming it or disrupting the harmony of its natural home.

Here I've illustrated three individual circumstances regarding confronting a pearl-embedded oyster, each with a different outcome. What was the variable? *Viewpoints*. We all have many, and there are as many collections of viewpoints as there are people. There are group viewpoints on some subjects, but I have never met two people who agree on everything, have you?

So, who is right? Is it possible then, that, on any given occasion, someone else who disagrees with me, when I *know* I'm right, can also be right? I think that my example bears this out. It is pretty common to observe well-intentioned people trying to label others, put them in categories, and file them away on a shelf in tidy little boxes. It may work with many things, but you can't pin down people or viewpoints and expect to lock them into groups by nationality, race, color, political, or sexual preferences.

One viewpoint is that if you look on the bright side of things, you are unrealistic. The late Earl Nightingale, famed motivator, was known to challenge people who called him a "Pollyanna" because of his positive views. He asked, "What makes a negative viewpoint more realistic than a positive one?"

Consider, if you will, that our planet is traveling through space at dizzying speeds and has been doing so for many millions of years without colliding with another planet or solar system. This is reality. It is also miraculous.

How about our sun. It is a ball of exploding gasses that burn day and night, without affecting us with a major variation of temperature, and has been doing so for millions of years. Then there is the human body with its sound system; tool kit of arms, fingers, and hands; video system; central cooling system; fueling system; and cleansing, ventilating, and disposal systems, all rolled up in a flexible, self-regenerating coat of skin—complete with its own portable computer.

I suggest that there must be a hundred million miracles that have to occur before we even wake up and get out of bed in the morning! Tell me why there isn't more justification for being optimistic than pessimistic. With Earl I say, "Get real!" Still, I must concede that there are as many viewpoints on this subject as there are people; therefore, those who hold to negativity as their reality have a right to their belief—and the results that come from expecting everything to go wrong.

A number of years ago I saw an interview with an ex-thief that supports my reasoning. He said that muggers watch people go by, observing their body language. If someone was prone to be a victim, he would see it and choose to attack him or her. Those who walked confidently were safe *by virtue of their consciousness!*

The point I hope to share with these stories is that we all evolve differently and have made our life choices based on our individual experiences, past results, past teachers, and desire for change. I recommend that our new choices be based on possibilities that will nurture ourselves, our planet, and those whose lives we touch.

I wish you joy, love, empowerment, loving friends, and an oyster, or shall I say, a pearl of wisdom.

The Power Within

Did you ever watch an ant carrying something ten times his size in his mouth? The ant is on a mission. It is his purpose in life. He doesn't question his fate. He is not aware that he is one of the smallest creatures on earth. He doesn't waste his time with comparisons or self-pity. Included in his make up is everything he needs to be useful and successful. His entire life is dedicated to the well-being of the entire community. This *purpose* drives him relentlessly. He knows who he is, and the Power within him animates his existence. There is much we can learn from the ant.

Consider the apple seed. It doesn't look like much, but within the apple seed is the blueprint of an apple tree that will grow, stretch out its branches and roots, and, when its time is fulfilled, produce bushels of its luscious fruit, year in and year out. Now, an apple seed, at first glance, doesn't look very powerful, but the potential within the seed is amazing. When just a seedling, it will grow around a rock to get its roots to water and its leaves to sunlight. As it grows in size and strength, the rock that once was a formidable obstacle is easily pushed aside by the powerful roots as they slowly move toward their most advantageous placement for the grounding, protection, and nutrition of the tree.

Why do these "lesser" creations do so naturally that which many of us fret about year after year? Does the tree doubt its destiny or its place in the universe? Does the ant give up when its home has been wrecked? Maybe it is time for us, the so-called dominators of our planet, to recognize the *power within us*. Perhaps we spend too much energy cultivating doubt and fear, and not enough on trust and vision. We certainly need to consider this possibility.

I have heard it said that "Nothing is as powerful as an idea whose time has come." Mary Baker Eddy wrote in 1875, "The devotion of thought to an honest achievement makes the achievement possible." What we are speaking of here is *mind power*, possibilities, and potential.

Here is an example of how it works. I speak to my friends up north during the winter. They ask, "How's the weather down there?" I tell them how beautiful it is. They call me a "lucky so and so." I then tell them that "luck" has nothing to do with it. I didn't win a lifetime vacation in Florida; I made a choice. I paid the price and got the benefits, and drawbacks, of my decision. They choose to live where they are as well and can change their choice any time they want.

Choice is power. It puts us in the driver's seat. The important questions are, Where are we going? And, Why? It is great to have the power to choose at our fingertips, but without a plan or purpose, we create our lives randomly. Living by choice is better than living by default because we are not victims of the choices of others. However, we need to have purpose to make wise choices. But how do we learn what our purpose is?

Like the apple seed, we arrive here with a perfect intrinsic plan, an intent. The three-year-old concert pianists we sometimes see on television prove to us that we arrive with a purpose. Unlike these prodigies, we are not always as clear about our life's calling. Self-doubt usually interferes. Realization of the power within sets us free to follow our path.

Here's the good news: Everything we do on our way to our life's work is an extra bonus. It is our education and training. Life is about living, not getting; about being, not becoming. We never finish our schooling anyway. We can choose to enjoy all of life's possibilities along the way. We have many more options than the ant or apple tree, and that makes for a more abundant life.

Live! Love! Play! And when you find your heart you will realize that your treasure was always there. One more thought: "Our purpose on earth is to express love. LOVE IS THE POWER WITHIN!"

Part 3

Delving

*After a biographical interlude,
this lighthearted section teaches powerful
truths that help and heal -
from voices on high.*

What would happen...

if we described

our health

and well-being

in as much

detail and emotion

as we describe

our illnesses

and negative beliefs?

—Author Unknown

Pause and Muse with Me

This chapter represents a few valuable perspectives. I took the liberty of jumping in and out of literary form and simply allowed my mind to be unbridled and lyrical. Please join me in this experiment and allow yourself to be equally light and soft as you read this.

The next chapter, "Spiritual Healing," offers biographical background of, and explanations for, my beliefs; some academic, some deeply ingrained. May they point you toward your own revelations and healings that dwell within the depths of your mind, *The Kingdom Within.*

I offer this thought: *A healing is not an event where sick matter changes to healthy matter.* A healing is a realization that life derives itself from the realm of God's perfection, not from the enactments of the ego mind. (The ego mind is a term used to describe thinking that is based in fear.) *When perfect love is realized, external conditions give way to spiritual law—every time. This is The Law and it is yours to use.*

So, come fly with me...

Spiritual Healing

My parents had no religion. Neither one of them associated themselves with a church. My dad, Sam, was raised Catholic, although he wasn't knowledgeable about the teachings. During World War II, he was stationed in Wichita Falls, Texas, where he met my mom, Mozelle. Mom had attended a fundamental Christian church. As a child she had many questions. Her minister had more or less told her that she had no right to ask questions as these were matters of faith and not open to discussion, so she abandoned that religion.

Mom and Dad were married by a justice of the peace and Dad was subsequently shipped overseas. After seeing enemy fire, Sam decided to see a priest—just in case. When, during conversation, the priest found out that Dad was not married in the church, he told him that he could not partake of the church sacraments (including last rites). Sam ended his association with the church.

By the time I was six, my parents decided that I should have a religion, but which one? A Jewish business associate recommended Christian Science to my parents because he had embraced it. We all went. They liked it, but didn't know how seriously to take it. (Christian Scientists did not drink alcoholic beverages, smoke, or call upon medical science for healing; they relied one hundred percent upon God for their every need.) I, on the other hand, loved the Sunday school and required my parents to bring me back. They had a short meeting and then cleaned out the medicine cabinets, threw out Sam's cigars, and their liquor.

As a family we all prayed together for each other and, including my younger brother Steve, spent many years being our own physicians.

I learned much about the power of prayer and trust during that time in my life. I remember an incident where a 900-pound cylinder from a printing press dropped and crushed Sam's right index finger. He was rushed to the hospital. By the time the doctor examined it, Sam had calmed himself. He asked to leave. The doctor told him the dire consequences of not having it treated. He used his left hand to sign a release and went back to work. You can guess the end of the story: a perfect finger, no deformity, no pain, and complete freedom of movement.

We witnessed many wonderful proofs of God's care through the years and, through our intense appreciation, we wondered how many blessings of protection had occurred that we didn't even know about.

I have been alert to the thousands of miracles that people usually called "luck" or "coincidence" throughout my life. In Sunday school we would read Jesus' admonition to his followers to do the same works that he did. I took it seriously. I felt so discouraged at times because I couldn't effect the instantaneous healings that he admonished us to perform.

In my thirties, during a divorce, I felt spiritually void and had a "crisis." It was at this time that I wrote the poem "Freedom's Way." This was the beginning, though I knew it not, of a whole new paradigm in my life. My inspiration for the next ten years came mainly from reading Unity's *Daily Word*, Dale Carnegie, Wayne Dyer, and eventually Louise Hay, whose writings led me to Science of Mind, where Ernest Holmes' teachings brought the magic back into my life.

With this whole new perspective, I was joyful. It wasn't long until it was tested. I was diagnosed with throat cancer. A doctor told me that there was a 50/50 chance I'd never speak again. Me, the auctioneer! I am, and always was, a communicator. What would I do without a voice. For three months I practiced vocal silence, and what an experience that was for me! One can't take anything for granted. We are such marvelous organisms!

I conceded to radiation treatments, prayed as I always had in the past, and practiced visualizations each morning when I went in for treatment. I would see, in my mind's eye, healing waves of life, love, and peace flowing through my body as they radiated me. That was ten years ago.

Today I give talks, auction, and speak on the phone daily without fear of loss.

The best part is that I had a poor singing voice before; now I sing fairly well. I even purchased professional karaoke equipment and went out working at clubs, singing and hosting. When I hear the biblical phrase "All things are possible through God," I nod in silent approval.

Haven't we, all of us, at one time or another had our own private miracles? The mistake would be to write them off as mysteries or coincidences.

This is my finding from fifty years of study: Harmony is the law, not the exception; but like the law of electricity, it only works for us when we plug in. Whether consciously or unconsciously, when we use the Law it works. Healing is a state of lifting consciousness from fear and doubt to love and trust. Miracles are the natural result of a perfect Law. All that is required is a change of beliefs.

We can give up fear and doubt for love, peace, and joy. It is in one's own keeping and not somewhere outside of ourselves. We must find our truth and our connection by going inside to the God within. "Seek and ye shall find."

The Many Miracles

My most recent phase of learning began about four years ago. I was in dire need of something "new," as I was reading the same things, in different books, over and over. It seemed that I had heard it all. I just wished I could perfect it. Why was I not seeing, in my current life, the sudden healings that Jesus demonstrated? Yes, I was manifesting greater good daily, and for this I was grateful, but I knew that there was more for me to do.

A close friend, Valerie, told me of a teacher whose integrity she trusted implicitly. Would I join them in attending weekly classes? I stopped what I was doing, although heavily invested monetarily and otherwise, and attended metaphysical classes conducted from a different vantage point. I learned about Universal Life Force, the energetic body, and how to move this healing energy by means of thought, breath, and the laying on of hands. Before this, everything I did spiritually was purely mental. Now I could experience spiritual occurrences in my body as well! *The moment I felt Life Force Energy in my hands, I knew that I had touched the Divine...and it had touched me back!*

I was taught to scan the aura and feel its energy. I never knew that people could see or feel anything that is unseen by the physical senses. I usually do not see the auric body, but have seen it on occasion, briefly. I do, however, feel it and receive guidance about it. To illustrate this guidance I offer the following story.

I was listening to Linda, the instructor, one evening, and sat behind a student, Michelle, who was obviously suffering with sinus congestion. My right hand suddenly rose from my lap with my palm pointed at the sufferer's head. I was amazed! I felt the Life Force Energy flowing through me and out from my hand to her. Without a word, Valerie and I reached out our hands simultaneously toward each other and grasped so that we formed a chain of energy flowing through her (on my left), through me, and out my right hand. A third student, Sue, joined in. No one said a word to each other or Michelle. Only a few minutes later, Michelle, startled by her suddenly clear head, turned to me, looked me in the eye, and exclaimed, "My head is clear! I'm healed. Thank you."

I sat there in shock. Who or what was working through me, and what part in this, if any, did I actually have? How did Michelle know what was going on behind her head? I still don't actually know.

I have heard from many that we have angels or guides that assist us. Usually, it is just in the form of a word or thought. In the next story it manifested as a physical impulse.

Bob was riding his motorcycle and was run off the road into a field, under a barbed wire fence. He felt a "hand" on his head, pushing it down, and then heard the sound of the barbed wire striking the top of his helmet. Had he not "ducked," he could have been beheaded. Bob told me that he believes in angels.

My experience is that I hear voices sharing information when I need it. Is it God? Angels? Guides? My own mind? I don't know. It is good, and it is there for me when I open myself to it. My belief is that there is always an answer and that it will be there when I need it, regardless of whose name I give to it.

As a result of the class, I experimented working with energy upon anyone who would let me. Many headaches were cleared, upset stomachs settled, and even arthritic pain relieved. OK, so the lame didn't walk, the blind see, or the dead rise, but I was being true to my soul and I experienced great joy that my touch had assisted these people to self-heal.

I immediately began systematically taking all the steps, one by one, to become a Reiki master. Reiki is an ancient Tibetan healing art that has had renewal since the early twentieth century in

Japan. It is one of many disciplines that I have studied in pursuit of a higher understanding.

I then had to determine what was happening when I was treating people. At the time of this writing, it is my belief that bringing people to stillness and allowing the unseen energies resident within each of us (Universal Life Force Energy) to balance each of us permits the body to heal itself. We don't actually "heal" anybody, but we can facilitate bringing the subject to a place where their intrinsic perfection reigns. Conditions are at best temporal, and if we are willing, we can release them. The Truth of God's power within each of us can then shine through—and *nothing happens*. That is, we see that we were always fundamentally pure and perfect spirit, only now it shows. So it is my opinion that we are not healers, but facilitators when we bring someone to the Truth that always was. I call this process "Nurturing the Soul" because I claim not to be a healer, but an allower and caregiver.

I'd like to share a very special story of what happened in my experience last spring. I call my story *The Rose...*

I received a call from my friend, Judy, telling me that Mary was in the hospital dying of cancer. She asked me to pray for her. I agreed. I hardly knew Mary, although she was well known by most of my friends. It's just that she and I had never spoken one on one except to exchange greetings. A few days later I received another call from

Glenna, who had moved to Arizona. She also asked me to pray for Mary. They really had my attention, so I called my Reiki friends, Valerie and Betsy, and we converged on the nursing home the Saturday before Easter.

We were all a little concerned because—well, you know how people can look during their final days with cancer. To our pleasant surprise, Mary lay asleep looking lovely, in fact, angelic. We all had brought a gift. There was an Easter basket and a bouquet; and I brought a single rose bud.

Mary seemed pretty well drugged and didn't stay conscious much, so we sat there practicing Reiki and praying for her.

At one point her roommate, who was obviously disturbed from her disease, came in agitated and making accusations. Mary rolled up, her back to me, appearing upset. I whispered, "Mary, do you want us to go?"

Mary turned 180 degrees, looked me in the eyes, and said, "No, I want to go!" She then closed her eyes again.

I took her rosebud in my hand and gently caressed her face with it. As I did, I told her that she had the freedom to make whatever choices she wanted. She could move into the light or stay here and fight it out on earthly terms. Either way, we would support her and God would be with her.

She opened her eyes, said "Thank you," and went back to sleep. *It was then that I looked at the rose. It was no longer a bud but a full-bloomed, wide-open rose.*

I don't know if I'll ever be able to explain what happened, but the laws of horticulture had just accelerated before our very eyes.

Mary awoke soon thereafter, and we all went for a walk. We sang the "Peace Song" and smiled together.

We left Mary knowing that she had given us more than we had brought her. A few days later she made her choice to go. Thanks, Mary, for your gifts.

Contemplation

When quiet moments finally overtake
  the harshness of the day and
  moonbeams replace traffic lights,
  I ask myself:
  Who am I?
  Why am I here?
  Shouldn't I be doing something?

As day after day races past me
  and my life flees like a rabbit
  freed from its cage, I wonder:
  What is worthy of my time?
  I seem to have so little.
  What do I value?
  What thief steals in the night
  my richest treasure, my life?
  And another day dawns
  and off I race.

I sit and write checks to pay for
  services and goods already
  received, but then halt because
  although the bills flow like the
  incoming tide, the numbers in my
  little checkbook deplete.
  I wonder if I am in control
  or just a lost soul.

The world around me slumbers as
I lie awake watching those same
moonbeams bounce on the pond
outside my window and dream
of a gentler way. A world where
life has value and joy.

And so I reach deep within
to that place where infinite
wisdom resides to ask,
"Father/Mother God,
Creator and Source of all life
and intelligence, tell me, I pray,
how do I live my life
wisely and usefully that I may not
reach the end of my days in
regret and shame, for I fear that
is where my life is going."

As I lie there in silence, I can feel
the gentle breeze from the
wings of the angels that watch
over me. Soft voices in the
stillness of my mind speaking
words of love and encouragement.
*"YOU MUST MASTER YOUR OWN
MIND. THERE IS NOTHING MORE
IMPORTANT FOR YOU TO DO HERE."*

"How do I do that?" I ask.

*"YOU MUST LIVE FROM A PLACE
OF WISDOM, TRUST, AND LOVE.
YOU MUST BANISH FEAR.
EVERY MOTIVE MUST BE UNITY WITH
YOUR SOURCE AND ALL LIFE.
NOTHING LESS IS WORTHY OF
A SOUL."*

"And how do I start?"

*"BEGIN NOW. I WILL SPEAK, YOU
WRITE. LEARN IN SILENCE, BUILD
CHARACTER IN THE STREAM OF
LIFE, WHERE YOU CAN FACE
YOUR OWN FOOLISHNESS
DISGUISED AS ANOTHER'S DEEDS.*

*"YOU MUST LEARN TO BE LOVE
IN ACTION."*

"Wow," thought I. "Answers from
angels; wisdom on wings. I shall
write of love and life and
purpose. I shall know where I
am going and why! Ah, Merciful
Father/Mother, teach me to live
love. I am ready."

Here is the wisdom that flowed
from heaven to this humble man...

PRAISE HEAVEN AND EARTH
  AND ALL THEREIN.
  WE NEED TO BE SAVED...
  FROM OUR OWN FEARS AND
  NOTHING ELSE!
  WE NEED ONLY TWO TOOLS
  FOR COMPLETE SUCCESS...
  A LOVING HEART AND A
  PEACEFUL, WILLING MIND.

  ALWAYS REMEMBER:
  IN THE GAME OF LIFE, WHO
  LOVES THE MOST—WINS.

Read on. The adventure continues.

Energy and Consciousness

All things are One.
    There is creator and creation,
    One.
    There is Life and Intelligence,
    One.
    There is Love and Law,
    One.
    There is black and white,
    One.
    There is male and female,
    One.
    There is Energy and Consciousness,
    One.
    One Universe, One People whose
    Source is the only One, the
    All There Is.

We will speak of the Spirit with
    words that are practical, lest
    we become so etheric that we
    lose ourselves in the clouds.

There are absolutes and relatives.
    Absolutes are unseen and
    unchangeable. Relatives are
    viewed physically, subject to
    our perceptions and have their

reality compromised by our
belief systems.

Reality is so powerful that we
need not subject that which is
seen to the unseen, for the unseen
and the visible are both real and
indestructible. Only the illusion
dies. The reality it symbolizes
continues. Both are necessary.

Release all *used to be*'s and open
your mind to the wonder of
what could be.

Expand Your Viewpoint

God: Law, Mind (wisdom and
intelligence), Life, Soul or Spirit,
Truth, Source (Father/Mother),
One, All there is. *God is Love*.
All of these words are
interchangeable. There is no
antonym in reality because
there is no other Life nor Power.
God is not only what man sees,
but also the Source of all reality.
Reality is invisible to limited
belief. The illusions of evil,
disease, and death vanish in the
light of Truth, the Truth that God
is All and we are made of the
only building block there is—this
same Origin and Cause—God.

Energy: *Light* vibrates, *sound*
vibrates, *thought* vibrates, atoms
and so-called matter vibrate. An
atom is made of space, some
electrons which are magnetic
impulses (feminine and attracting),
offset by some protons
(masculine, radiant)...and
transparent neutrons.

We now surmise all form to be
vibration perceptible by our physical and
spiritual senses. We, ourselves, are pure
energy and live in an energy world...
Einstein's *Unified Field*.
Energy is Intelligence.
It is the source of all life.
It is the essence of *All There Is*.
Many of us call it Universal Life
Force. It is pliable by thought,
and is the building block of
consciousness.

Consciousness: Universal Intelligence.
In relative terms, it is a way of
thinking, a mindset. Consciousness
is how and where we create the
world in which we live. Because
there are as many relative truths
as there are people, *no two
people live in the same world*.
In absolute terms, consciousness
is where we "live and move and
have our being." Consciousness is
All There Is.

Our Task: To evolve our relative
consciousness back to the Original
Consciousness through love and

trust. This means loving our way back to reality. We can evolve no farther than our *lowest* estimation of our fellow man. To the degree we see perfection in all life, to that degree do we raise our consciousness to a place of love.

The Obstacles: A belief in separatism...
That God is distant, instead of being our very lives.
That we are better or worse than others.
That there is a power to oppose All There Is.
That we are inadequate to live our lives and make intelligent choices.
That we need the approval of someone else to be valuable.
That we are powerless.
That God is powerless.

All of these obstacles are a form of illusion. Our objective need be only this:
TO LOVE AND TRUST MORE EACH DAY.
This would raise the vibration of our relative consciousness so that we resonate with spiritual harmony.

In this Truth lies all healing,
growth, peace, and happiness.

When we hate, fear, and doubt,
  we restrict our upward path to that
  place of perfection from which we
  originated.
  The objective is to be of One Mind
  with the Universe and thereby bring
  heaven (harmony) to earth
  (visibility). The obstacles are many,
  but they are powerless. They are
  subject to our choices.

An Important Reminder

WE ARE HERE TO BE HAPPY.
   TO LIVE, LOVE, AND REJOICE
   IN THE GLORY OF GOD'S LOVE.
   WE ARE HERE TO VIEW, WITH
   AWE, THE VASTNESS OF
   CREATION.

THE WORLD WITH ITS HARDSHIPS IS
   A MYTH, AN ILLUSION.
   IF WE ARE TO DISPEL THIS
   DREAM WORLD, WE MUST LEARN
   TO PLAY.
   SMILE! GIVE UP FEAR FOR
   THANKSGIVING.
   GIVE UP WORRY AND DOUBT FOR
   ENTHUSIASM AND TRUST.
   GIVE UP YOUR CONTROLS AND
   BE FREE. LET GO!

My friend, Joan, sent me the following
   answer to worry and fear.

Good morning, Dear One. This is God.
I will be handling all your problems
   today.
I will not need your help.
So let's go out and have a wonderful day.
—Earthly Author Unknown

Part 4

The Tools

Discover the blocks that are holding you back. Then use the tools in this section to dissolve them.

Do not feel

totally, personally,

irrevocably

responsible for

everything...

that is my job!

—God

—Author Unknown

Designing a Life

So you want to design a new life. You've pushed and tugged and fought and prayed and still it all seems to remain beyond your reach.

That could be why! The need for control, making things go *your* way, is NOT the answer. We don't need to be in control. Let go! What is needed is simple trust.

No matter how much I pray, meditate, read, contemplate, or think, the answer that comes to me is always the same: "Let go, observe, and trust a perfect outcome."

Does this mean make no plans? No. Does it mean have no desires? No. Does it mean let other people run your life? No. What it does mean is to let your intuition lead you and observe the way things are evolving. I have a note on my desk that came off the internet somewhere: "Make God your partner and success will follow."

This is a simple but difficult lesson. We continue to think that if we let go, we will fall and hurt ourselves, so we hang on to the controls until our muscles ache and our vision blurs. This does not control anything. The earth is still traveling at astronomical speeds, and our lives are passing us like lightning. There is nothing we own and almost nothing we can control.

We can, however, choose our thoughts, and herein lies the only area we can direct. This is where we must start and finish our life's journey. If we find that smiling brings us a feeling of inner peace, we must smile often. If we find that breathing deeply relaxes us, we must pause and deep breathe periodically. These are mechanisms that serve us. If loving and blessing bring us happiness, we must love and bless with reckless abandon. If giving appreciation empowers us and those we recognize, we must lavish praise and appreciation upon ourselves and them, as often and sincerely as possible.

On the other hand, if we are immobilized, we are in fear. If we are confused, we are in fear. If we are angry, we are in fear. If we are hating, we are fearing. If we doubt, we are being fearful. If we are discouraged, in pain, in illness, or whatever distress, it is only fear wearing a different disguise. A pattern is emerging here.

Observe. As you watch you will see that *the belief in our separation from a perfect and loving God creates fear.* Accept that premise and suffer. The consequences of believing in a world of separate little beings, alone and afraid, open the door to all the ills, despondency, and pain man chooses to endure.

The remedy? Love, forgiveness, gratitude, and trust. Trust that the Universe supports you. Trust that the "will of God" (God's Law) is good. Universal Law is love and peace and a perfect, orderly path. To get on this path and experience the joy that awaits REQUIRES you to:

- *Let go of the reigns and trust a perfect outcome.*
- *Take each moment and live it to the fullest.*
- *Seek out ways to share love and happiness.*
- *GIVE UP THE NEED TO ALWAYS BE RIGHT.*
- *Allow the energy or spirit of Life to flow through you, and feel the peace and harmony that is inherent in this attitude.*

HAPPINESS IS ABOUT ATTITUDES.
PEACE IS ABOUT LOVE AND TRUST.

Tools for Building a Powerful Future

We all have learned to work with certain tools. This is a concept that is common to all of us. Whether we be household engineers (formerly called housewives during the unenlightened era), construction workers, office personnel, fishermen, healers, or whatever, we all own and use tools. In the office it might be a computer. For repairs we can use test equipment and wrenches. The human body arrived here with tools: a brain for processing information with more competency than any man-made computer; hands that can do more functions than any mechanical tool ever devised; eyes, ears, and a nose to be used as test equipment and for directional guidance; legs and feet to take us where we want to go; and a chemical pharmacy that delivers on demand! Our body is a wondrous machine, and those of us who have studied its systems can't help being in awe of the intelligence of the designer of its systems.

Yet our body is not our greatest tool. No, the body is a mere lump without receiving direction. It is the mind that wins the prize as the Greatest Tool of All. Not the brain, an organ that sorts and files and runs programs. I'm speaking of the thinker who directs the brain and body—the mind that creates our lives and experiences and chooses meaning to attribute to all of the events of our lives. It is you, the thinker, that I am addressing. Your beliefs and attitudes determine your quality of life. It has been proven over and over again that the mind can rise above the seeming limitations of the body taking us to astounding heights.

Next, let's do something I don't often do. Let's intentionally talk about *negative tools* or *programs* (blocks). We can talk them up, put them down, and, hopefully, replace them with *positive tools*.

Negative Tools (The Blocks)

1. Disempowerment: Making others wrong so that we can make ourselves right.

How subtle is the error of thinking that we must be "right." What is required to think that our opinion is law and others must do things our way? A frail ego that cannot bear the thought of being "wrong." We feel so imperiled at the thought of not being right, of being "bad" or "foolish." We are terrorized by this notion and lash out at others, making them feel wrong so we can go back to the illusory safety of being right. This is *all about judgmentalism, not judgment. Consider the harm we can provide others and ourselves through disempowerment.*

2. Doubt: Distrusting the Universe.

Doubt never created a useful result. Doubting others' versions of fiction can be helpful, but doubt, of itself, only discredits. It has no other merit. Doubt is fear-based, a belief that we are not good enough for things to work out beautifully, an attitude of surrender to inevitable failure. It is a Godless belief and unsuitable for spiritual or even human growth. *No progress ever came from doubting the infinite possibilities.*

3. Discouragement: The wedge. The belief that all is hopeless, that the present difficult moment represents the entirety of life.

Let me explain the wedge. There is an old fable called *The Devil's Auction*. It seems that spending in hell had gotten so badly out of hand that the Devil was forced to auction off his tools. One very courageous farmer who had watched the proceedings for quite some time walked over to an ever-smiling Satan and remarked, "I have watched some very heavy bidding for lust, greed, and resentment. Yet you seem not very concerned at all by their loss. In the glass case you are leaning against is a hand-carved wedge with a 'Not for Sale' sign on it. May I ask why you look so happy?"

The Devil replied, "Sure. The sale is going well and I am bringing in big money. That is important to me. People are fighting and getting angry out of fear that they won't get their prize. I enjoy watching that. The wedge you asked about is my prize tool. It is not for sale because it is the only one I need to accomplish my end. It succeeds where other tools fail. If I want to acquire peoples' souls, they must first give up. The wedge is *discouragement*, and it is remarkably useful for the end I desire."

The moral of this story is: *Never give up!!!*

4. Guilt: A purposeless, useless emotion based upon fear of having been wrong in the past.

Guilt is debilitating. It tells you that you are wrong and that your personal worth is low because you have made a mistake. Guilt implies that you are not deserving of anything good. Like all negative tools, it relies upon a belief in separation from the Divine Source. It separates you from your friends, family, or associates and prevents you from the accomplishment of your dreams; yet this is why you are here! To live your dreams and the loving interaction of your relationship with God, man, and nature. Operating out of guilt is a painful mistake. Turn the past over to God and trust a perfect outcome.

5. Worry: Nervous doubt. *The opposite process of thinking.* Don't confuse worry with concern. Concern would indicate that you are considering possible consequences in an attempt to make a deliberate, intelligent choice. Worry has no rationale. It is fear of the future and also the unknown. Worry presumes that we are frail, defective, and defenseless. When we worry, we imagine unhappy results. It is often guilt-based. Fear of the future, based upon unsatisfactory past results, inadequacy, or lack of self-esteem, is the basis for worry.

Worry dissipates when we have a plan. A plan constitutes an expectation of greater possibilities. We can leave the future and past to be here and now. Taking positive forward steps redeems us from the immobility of fear or worry.

It is difficult, if not impossible, to worry when we are living in the now. Worry kicks in as soon as we think about *later*.

6. Self-depreciation: This is not humbleness. It is rejecting our spiritual gifts as *not good enough*. This tool protects us from looking conceited and thereby being unlovable. We were taught as children to not let our good appearance, our intelligence, or our accomplishments go to our heads. This was good advice. All good things should be removed from the *head* and inserted directly into the *heart*, where they can do the most good!

7. Control: Manipulating people and events out of pure fear. Most of us want to feel that we are in control. We wouldn't start up our car, put it in gear, and let it drive us to work while we go back to sleep, because we know we wouldn't get far before there would be repercussions. Therefore, we have decided that to be in control of our own destiny is the right thing. This is correct. It is when we decide that we must control other people, so that we can be in control of our own lives, that we get into trouble. Control is so subtle sometimes that we don't realize it. Other times we know that we are controlling others, but we override this because we decide that it is in their own best interest, or ours, or someone else's. We have at this point overstepped. Personal boundaries become thin when we care about others; but make no mistake, we are biting off too much when we make other peoples' decisions for them.

Eventually we must come to a place in our lives where we offer our kindest thoughts, remove ourselves lovingly, and then *let go and let God* handle the details.

8. Comparison: The main source of discontent. Although comparing results may help us make wiser decisions at times, trusting our intuition works better. Comparing our lives to others' and feeling downtrodden because we have not done as well is a huge mistake. First of all, we really do not know what all of the circumstances are in another's experience. Secondly, we are always our own worst critics. Seldom do we realize how well we really are doing. Occasionally, we will receive an amazing compliment from a friend showing admiration for our character, wisdom, or style. Usually we give away such "flattery" as uninformed. We are better served to take special note of this information. We need to learn our strengths. Most of us spend far too much energy agonizing over our "shortcomings." *No two lives are identical, and, therefore, they are not comparable.*

In school we were taught that we must "measure up" in academic grading and sports competition. This falsely inflated a few people and grossly affected the self-esteem of most of the rest. So, instead of brow-beating ourselves or other people for not measuring up, we can get out another yardstick and take another look. Everyone has his/her own gifts, and we err by counting their gifts and discounting our own. First cash in your own chips before you decide everyone else has more than you do. Have you really lived your potential completely? If not, don't fold your hand. Get back in the game and bet everything on your own ability to live a rich, happy life!

9. Three more C's: Criticism, Complaint, and Condemnation (judgmentalism).

There is nothing we can do that is more destructive than to criticize. It single-handedly has undone all of the benefits of the perfect life we received at birth. As soon as people began telling us that we were bad, wrong, foolish or stupid, life went downhill.

Then there were the inferences that we were inadequate. Kids can be especially cruel, teasing, and taunting. They learn the process from adults and practice Criticism without restraint. It can take a colossal effort, over a period of many years, to break down these stigmas in our minds, a demoralization started soon after birth. Seldom do people get over the damage from this negative tool.

Complaint destroys the joy of the complainer and the recipient. We all know how unpleasant it is to spend time with complainers. Tell someone about a complaint you have and a dozen more people will jump in with their complaints. Commiseration is a favorite pastime of people in like circumstances. Healing and joy don't arise from these conversations.

Condemnation is a very strong word. We associate it with another "C" word, Censure. We don't realize that we condemn someone every time we say, "He always does that..." or "She can't help herself." To condemn is to say "always" or "never" about people, making it clear that they will be in a negative state—forever. *We must not label any person or group*. In doing that, we have mentally sentenced them and closed our own mind, which equates to lovelessness. A loving, open mind, with expectation of continual unfoldment and spiritual growth, is required by all of us, sooner or later.

Consider this adjustment in thought and attitude now: The world can rise, in your experience, no higher than your belief about it. Give the world lots of love if you want to participate in spiritual change for everyone. We can and must change our attitudes and open our hearts. The time has come for us to be more, receive more, give more, and expect more.

10. Blame: Accusation, a great way to give away your power! Blaming others pays dividends. You don't have to take responsibility or make any changes; you just get to make someone else feel bad. Blame is vicious criticism, and you already know the fruitage of such thinking.

Positive Tools

1. Love: Here is a subject that could not be covered in its entirety. If all of the writings and volumes ever written on the subject were compiled, and it would be a massive collection, there still would not be an adequate explanation. Let me then simply say that, above all else, there is love. It is the life and substance of *All There Is*; the Creator and the Total Creation; consciousness and energy expressed as kind gestures, appreciation, gratitude, joy, nurturing (and self-nurturing), power, and unity; the opposite of fear; the universal magnet or attractor; the only gift that is truly worthy to give to God and God's children. Use love as your tool to move mountains, still the fear of a brother or sister, or to motivate your life. Nothing less is worthy of a life's work.

2. Gratitude: The open door to supply. Joyful appreciation of the Divine Source and all of Its expressions. The antidote for criticism, complaint, and judgmentalism. The attitude that heals resentment and pain. You cannot be grateful and unhappy at the same time, so pick one.

3. Appreciation and praise: Love in relationship to people and life. An attitude that can turn any life from failure to success. What makes someone prosperous or poor is *not* money. It is an attitude of appreciation for all things big and small. It is finding happiness while others manage to find misery in the same places. Appreciation and praise for others can turn lives around. People are so starved for appreciation that a word of praise is liable to open a floodgate of tears. With the common experience of criticism and judgmentalism facing us at every intersection of life, it is so powerful to share these wonderful tools. You will find yourself swamped with devoted friends and supporters if you can open yourself earnestly to dispense kindnesses by merely appreciating that which really is good in those you encounter, and genuinely praising them for their special characteristics. I will preach this with my last breath: To give love during this lifetime in the most powerful path available; feel appreciation and give praise.

4. Trust: The tool to overturn control, doubt, and discouragement. When we teach children to swim or ride a bicycle, we must at some point let them go. These are trust issues on the part of both parent and child. When we are trusting we are not controlling. We don't need to be assured of a particular outcome. The reward is the trusting itself. Letting go is so freeing that our health instantly improves.

Doubts would make us crazy. It was pointed out to me: When we mail a letter, we drop it in the box and forget about it. We don't park and wait for the mail truck to come pick it up. We don't follow the truck to the airport or catch a flight to make sure that it arrived safely. We simply let go and trust its arrival. We are seldom disappointed. We are always freed by letting go. There is a perfect law and a perfect plan. For these to work in one's life, one must let go and trust.

5. Affirmations: Tools for building a consciousness that can manifest our every need, any time, any place. What we lack, aside from trust, in many cases is conviction. Conviction arises from repeated experiments that demonstrate a reliable principle. Affirmations are one of several powerful techniques for making things in our life go well. Motivators call this "positive self-talk." When we speak our truth we give it life. We create thought-forms. The Creator created the entire universe, we are told, with a word. We, as co-creators, can do the same thing. We affirm a positive outcome to a negative situation. We release our declarations with trust and expectancy. All of a sudden there is a shift in circumstances and the problem has mysteriously resolved itself. This can be more than an experiment; it can be a way of life.

Affirmations must always be positive. For instance, "My business won't fail" is not an affirmation. It creates a plausibility of failure. "My business grows stronger each day" as an affirmation can build a mighty empire from a tiny idea.

The other thing to know is that affirmations must be spoken or written in the present. "My business will grow stronger" puts off the manifestation to an unknown tomorrow. "My business grows stronger each day" starts now. Keep your affirmations in the now. Expect to see changes. Don't stop affirming. It is a wonderful way of life and frees you to plant the seeds and move on. Unfoldment comes in the way Spirit chooses, and it is most often much better than anything you could have planned if you tried! Affirmations work wonders. Try them and see for yourself.

6. Visualization: What the mind sees, it believes and reproduces. In my story, "Creating a Better World," in Part 2, I gave an example of how, through visualization, I turned a fiasco into a dream come true. We must learn to see beyond the evidence of the five fallacious physical senses. The facts of the senses turn to fictitious memories when the power of the mind is applied. It was ever thus and ever will be.

To use this mighty tool, begin by practicing visualizing what it would be like to have something you desire very much. I don't mean, "I see my ex-girlfriend taking me back..." because that imposes your will on another and Universal Law won't permit the interference in another's free will. If a love relationship was your need, instead visualize yourself walking along the beach or wherever you'd want to be with a wonderful mate.

Create the partner's character and qualities. Especially visualize a partner who blends with your life, who loves and nurtures you in a way you've never been loved before.

Picture every minute detail. Hold in your mind's eye the joy; feel it, smell it, taste it. Open your heart to the possibility and a miracle is on its way. A word of caution. Don't overlook anything that is important to you. Don't generalize. Don't settle. You will manifest. Make sure you get what you really want. If you specify, for instance, a rich person, you might have to deal with all the benefits *and limitations* of people who live for money. You might use a better phrase like "with a healthy financial attitude and source of supply" so that your mate shows up and is not stingy or doesn't use money to manipulate you.

Visualization works. Don't neglect this powerful tool for creating anything your heart truly desires.

7. Prayer and meditation: Scientific tests have proved the efficacy of both of these tools. There are as many ways to pray and meditate as there are teachers and disciples. For me, prayer is talking (usually affirming) and meditation is listening.

Some sit repeating a mantra for hours. Others listen to meditation tapes with soft voices, music, or subliminal messages behind the sound of ocean waves. Some people get on their hands and knees and beg God to help them. Some surrender their fears and doubts to an omnipotent Creator. I write letters to God and wait for the answers. This is asking and listening, and it seems to work exceptionally well when I quietly tune in.

The list of ways is endless. If you have no pattern established, or if you are stuck in one that is not fruitful for you, I suggest that you try different ways until something feels right—and works for you. Do remember that if you ask, answers will somehow come. They may come in dreams or flashes of brilliance, in visions, or just an inner knowing. It does not matter. Put time aside daily to ask and listen. Have a preprogrammed plan for the session. Start by following your plan. After that, be still and let Spirit take you wherever it wants. Infinite Intelligence knows better than you or I anyway.

Larry Dossey has written several books based on the scientific testing of the efficacy of prayer to bring about change. He made it clear that he was not writing about religion, merely the intent of people to entreat on behalf of others. The results in these double-blind tests were astonishing to the scientific world, if not to those who hold these loving intentions for others as a way of life.

You can't do it wrong. I repeat: *You can't do it wrong*. Don't let form inhibit you. Spirit will talk to your soul. Show up and listen.

Energy

I am a Reiki master. I have studied the Silva Method, Joh Rei, Pranic Healing, Triple Helix, Therapeutic Touch, and Healing Touch. I have taken weekend seminars with Barbara Brennan and Carolyn Myss. My revelation from all this is: "*Energy is All There Is*." The Japanese call it *ki*, the Chinese call it *chi*, and the Indians call it *prana*. Energy or Universal Life Force is that which constitutes all life and expression. Its substance is pure love, and it changes the illusion of material conditions whether applied by thought, breath, sound, smell, or by the laying on of hands.

An excellent text on the form and nature of energy and the human energy field is presented in Barbara Brennan's book, *Hands of Light*. James Redfield's *Celestine Prophesy* is perhaps the easiest way to become acquainted with the subtle, nonphysical energies. I just want to say that energy can be transformed but never destroyed, so by learning of the Universal Life Force (that which is around you, within you, and fills all space...that which unifies all mankind, life, and creation), we enhance our skills of dealing with the spiritual realms from which we originated.

I welcome you to continue on your path of discovery with me. Let not this little book be your final text. It is my gift from a great deal of study. May it assist you on your journey toward finding your highest truths and greatest joys.

Purpose

Everyone has a purpose and needs a vision. Let your life be about your purpose, and you can't help blessing yourself and all whom you encounter. As an example, I present my vision. May it open your heart and empower you, right now, to create a new possibility, meaning, and purpose for your life.

You can do this by taking the time to decide what you want for the rest of your life, make it your dream and follow that dream. If you don't know what you want, you can't get it! This is the most important part of manifestation. Know who you are, decide what you want, DON'T ASSUME OTHERS KNOW. Hold your highest truths in consciousness and watch the universe fulfill your highest desires!

I bring my vision to reality through the power of my word. My word creates my truth, and my truth is a new order on planet earth. *My purpose is loving life and empowering others*. I see this empowerment as a long-awaited transformation from a prior place of unknowing and yearning into new possibilities. I envision those whom I bless (by acts of recognition, acceptance, gratitude, appreciation, and love) sharing a higher consciousness and bringing this energy into their own community.

I foresee community after community networking, growing, sharing, and giving as a way of life. When the point of critical mass is reached, and I expect it in my lifetime, I perceive a quantum leap in world consciousness. I envision the sudden and powerful reality of a world enthroned in love and peace—a planet once again covered with beautiful forests, clean air, and clear water.

All hunger, blame, guilt, and hatred will disappear. We will live in an unshackled world with no harmful beliefs remaining to inhibit its never-ending unfoldment.

I acknowledge this vision as true, here and now!

Amen: It is done.

Remember

Life is not linear, it is cyclical. We travel an upward spiral. Periodically, we find ourselves back where we started in most areas of our lives. Each Time, however, we are looking down from a brand new perspective. Through our trials and tribulations, we have grown. When we look at our world at the finish of a cycle, it is not the same world in which we started out. I make this point because this book becomes new each time I read it. It is a healing text for me. When life complicates, I read this book to find my heart once again. If I am not being joyful, I have let my head take over. In one's heart is the place where all joy exists.

If you found your joy in this book, go back to it when you're feeling beaten or defeated to rekindle your hope, gratitude, trust, wisdom, appreciation, love, enthusiasm and power. The words, ideas, and concepts will become yours for all time and will carry you through the deepest waters and harshest storms as they have for me. It has been said that knowledge is power. I add to this, knowledge of Spiritual Truth, the understanding of the Universal Life, Intelligence, Love and Law which created us and sustain us, is the only true and eternal power. Let this be the truth that empowers your life, live in this consciousness and rejoice forevermore!

My Appreciation

Thank you, dear reader, for taking the time to read the product of my half-century of study and contemplation. I suspect that, by now, you are clearly aware that your life is pure potential and that you can tap into this power source to make the wise choices that will enable your life to soar.

As the Dream Maker said, *"Discipline is the element you must add to Wisdom, Faith, and Love to make them a day-to-day reality...it is certainly the part of the job you must accomplish for yourself."*

I implore you to take action. Don't stop here! Please join me and a multitude of lightworkers in our unified purpose of bringing peace, love, and beauty back to planet earth by offering your prayers, meditations, visualizations, and daily acts of kindness.

We have entered together a new age of spiritual consciousness and power. Let this little book assist you on your journey. Share it with those you love. Share your love with the people you meet at work, at home, at recreation, and on the highway in between. Let the meaning of your life be the love you are living. My blessings go with you.

"The End"
of this book.
"The Beginning"
of our journey together as lightworkers.

You can visit the author anytime at
http://www.wisdom and healing.com

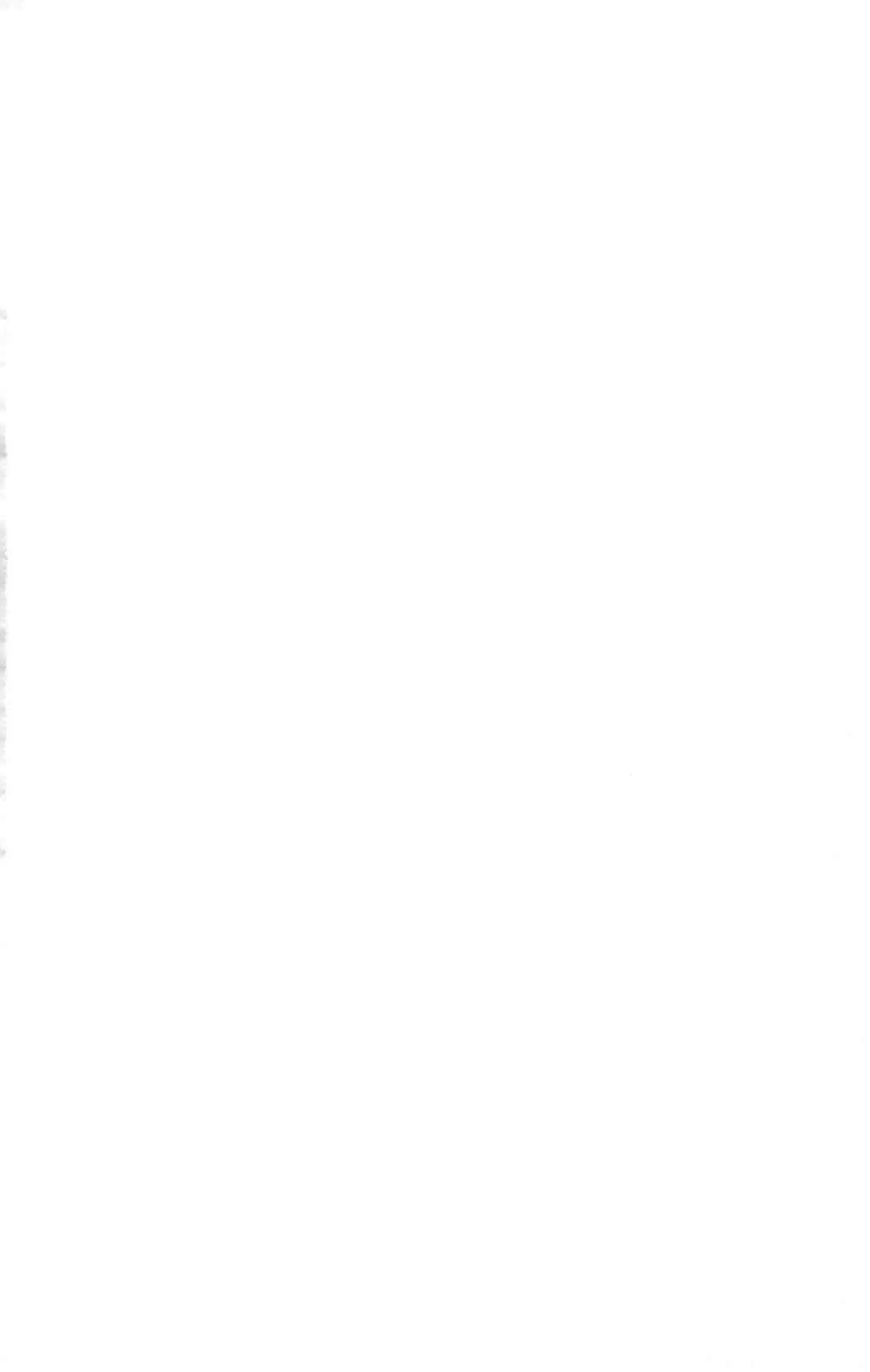